Study Guide for

Health Psychology
An Introduction to Behavior and Health

Fourth Edition

Study Guide for

Health Psychology
An Introduction to Behavior and Health

Fourth Edition

Linda Brannon

Jess Feist

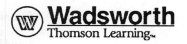

Wadsworth
Thomson Learning™

Australia • Canada • Denmark • Japan • Mexico • New Zealand • Philippines
Puerto Rico • Singapore • South Africa • Spain • United Kingdom • United States

For permission to use material from this text,
contact us by
        Web: www.thomsonrights.com
        Fax: 1-800-730-2215
        Phone: 1-800-730-2214

For more information, contact
Wadsworth/Thomson Learning
10 Davis Drive
Belmont, CA 94002-3098
USA
www.wadsworth.com

International Headquarters
Thomson Learning
290 Harbor Drive, 2nd Floor
Stamford, CT 06902-7477
USA

UK/Europe/Middle East
Thomson Learning
Berkshire House
168-173 High Holborn
London WC1V 7AA
United Kingdom

Asia
Thomson Learning
60 Albert Complex
Singapore 189969

Canada
Nelson/Thomson Learning
1120 Birchmount Road
Scarborough, Ontario M1K 5G4
Canada

ISBN 0-534-36852-2

Contents

Preface

We have designed this Study Guide to accompany our *Health Psychology: Introduction to Behavior and Health* (4th ed.), and each chapter corresponds to a chapter in that text. Each of the seventeen chapters of the Study Guide is divided as follows:

- **Fill in the Rest of the Story** is a fill-in-the-blanks exercise that tests your ability to recall important terms, concepts, and definitions. Fill in the blanks and check your answers with those provided.

- **Multiple Choice Questions** allow you to test your recognition memory. Many of these items may be similar to those you will see on your quizzes and tests. Mark your answers and check their accuracy.

- A **Matching Exercise** appears in some chapters. This exercise is oriented toward pairing researchers or theorists with their work. Your instructor may refer to research by the names of those who did the study, and this matching exercise should help you attend to and absorb this information. This exercise appears in chapters that have many names that might confuse students.

- **Essay Questions** measure your ability to organize and present key points in each chapter. We have provided an extensive answer outline for each essay question to allow you to check not only information but also organization.

- **Let's Get Personal** is an individualized exercise that gives you an opportunity to integrate the health information in each chapter into your own life.

- **Visual Exercises** appear in some of the chapters and will challenge you to identify important information visually. These exercises are similar to figures in the text, and you should complete the figure by supplying the missing labels, and then checking the text for the correct answers.

We wish to acknowledge Patrick Moreno and to thank him for his help in preparing this Study Guide.

Purchasing the textbook and study guide are only a preliminary step toward mastering the course material in health psychology. Unfortunately, we have discovered no magical way to infuse knowledge or to make studying effortless. We designed the exercises in this study guide to give you a variety of approaches to learn health psychology, but none of these study devices will help if you do not use them. Reading the text and attending class are important in learning and in making good grades. We hope that you use this study guide to organize and assimilate the volume of information in health psychology. We believe that working through the study guide exercises can help you make better grades and can make health psychology part of your life.

Good luck in studying health psychology,

Linda Brannon

Jess Feist

Study Guide for

Health Psychology
An Introduction to Behavior and Health

Fourth Edition

CHAPTER 1
Introducing Health Psychology

Fill in the Rest of the Story

I. The Changing Field of Health

During the 20th century, the field of health changed because patterns of

illness changed. At the beginning of the century, most illness were

_____ and of short duration, and now most are

_____ and relate to behavior and lifestyle.

A. Patterns of Disease and Death

Currently, the two leading causes of death in the United States and other

industrialized countries are _____ _____ and

_____. These diseases affect old people more often than young

people. Teenagers and young adults are most likely to die of

_____ _____. Ethnic background is also a

factor in life expectancy, but poverty and _____ level relate to

ethnic background, making this factor difficult to determine.

B. Escalating Cost of Medical Care

The costs of medical care has risen more rapidly than _____,

leading some people to question the cost effectiveness of cures.

1

C. What Is Health?

Some people define health as freedom from illness, but health psychologists

prefer to define health as a _____ state; that is, a state of well-being.

D. Changing Models of Health

The biomedical model holds that disease is due to the presence of an outside

agent called a _____ that causes disease. An alternative model,

the _____ model, adds psychological and social factors to

biological ones, resulting in a more comprehensive view of health and illness.

II. Psychology's Involvement in Health

Psychology's involvement in health concentrates on _____

factors in the development of many chronic diseases. Health psychologists also

help people cope with stress, pain, and chronic illness.

A. Psychology in Medical Settings

Until the development of health psychology, psychologists who were involved

in medical training either taught in _____ school or provided

clinical consultation.

B. Psychosomatic Medicine

The view that physical illness has its roots in psychological and emotional

conflicts is called _____ medicine and has its roots in

_____ theory.

C. Behavioral Medicine

The interdisciplinary field that attempts to integrate behavioral and biomedical knowledge and techniques and which applies this knowledge to prevention, diagnosis, treatment, and rehabilitation is called

_____ _____.

D. Behavioral Health

Behavioral health focuses on _____ of illness and enhancement of health rather than on diagnosis, treatment, and rehabilitation.

E. Health Psychology

Health psychology is that field of psychology dealing with the scientific study of _____ that relate to health enhancement, prevention, and rehabilitation. Psychologists interested in health-related issues founded the psychological specialty of health psychology and formed Division 38 of the

_____ _____ Association.

Answers

I.   acute (infectious); chronic
I.A.   heart disease (cardiovascular disease); cancer; unintentional injuries (accidents); educational
I.B.   inflation
I.C.   positive
I.D.   pathogen; biopsychosocial model
II.   behavioral (lifestyle)
II.A. medical
II.B. psychosomatic; Freudian (psychoanalytic)
II.C. behavioral medicine
II.D. prevention
II.E. behaviors; American Psychological

Multiple Choice Questions

_____ 1. Which of these has been a major health trend in the United States since the beginning of the 20th century?
   a. Medical costs have risen faster than rate of inflation.
   b. The medical model has narrowed, concentrating more strongly on the biomedical model.
   c. Health was defined as the presence of positive well-being at the beginning of the century but is now defined as the absence of illness.
   d. Acute illnesses have replaced chronic diseases as the leading causes of death.

_____ 2. Diseases that develop and persist over a long period of time
   a. include influenza and pneumonia.
   b. are no longer the leading causes of death in the U. S.
   c. are called infectious diseases.
   d. are called chronic diseases.

_____ 3. About 19% of all deaths and the leading cause of preventable deaths in the Unites States are the result of
   a. use of tobacco products.
   b. improper diet.
   c. violence.
   d. sexual behaviors.

_____ 4. For young people in the United States ages 15 to 24, the leading cause of death is
   a. unintentional injuries.
   b. suicides.
   c. homicides.
   d. sexual behaviors.

_____ 5. Life expectancy in the United States has _____ since 1900.
   a. increased by about 20 years
   b. increased by about 30 years
   c. decreased by about 10 years
   d. remained about the same

_____ 6. The dramatic increase in life expectancy in the United States since 1900 is mostly the result of
   a. reduction in cardiovascular disease.
   b. increases in visits to health care providers.
   c. decreases in infant mortality.
   d. adults taking better care of themselves.

_____ 7. Which of these has contributed MOST to escalating medical costs?
   a. increased population
   b. decreases in chronic disease
   c. sophisticated medical technology and complex surgical procedures
   d. uninsured motorists

_____ 8. People whose beliefs are consistent with the biomedical model
   a. believe that health is a positive condition.
   b. think that they are healthy when they don't feel sick.
   c. believe that they are sick when others tell them that they are sick.
   d. believe that they can become healthy mostly through self treatment.

_____ 9. The biopsychosocial view of health is most likely to be held by
   a. health psychologists.
   b. the federal government.
   c. traditional medicine.
   d. people who see health as an ideal state.

_____ 10. Any agent that can cause a disease is called a(n)
   a. risk factor.
   b. illness.
   c. infection.
   d. pathogen.

_____ 11. The search for microscopic organisms that cause disease
   a. prevented the acceptance of the biomedical model.
   b. prevented significant medical progress during the 19th century.
   c. were the main cause of medical advances during the 19th century.
   d. both a and b

_____ 12. The person who argued that modern physicians have lost touch with the empathic bedside manner was
   a. G. Stone.
   b. J. Matarazzo.
   c. S. Freud
   d. H. F. Dunbar

_____ 13. Beau attributes his "cold" to not getting enough sleep and to recent stressful life experiences. Thus, it seems that Beau's beliefs are consistent with
   a. the biochemical model of health.
   b. the biomedical model of health.
   c. the biopsychosocial model of health.
   d   Cartesian dualism.

_____ 14. That aspect of medicine that views physical illnesses as having emotional and psychological components is called
   a. health psychology.
   b. behavioral health.
   c. Cartesian medicine.
   d. psychosomatic medicine.

_____ 15. Behavioral health emphasizes
   a. the importance of psychosomatic medicine.
   b. the prevention of illness and the enhancement of health.
   c. the treatment of disease.
   d. the importance of stress in chronic illnesses.

_____ 16. The discipline that focuses on the scientific study of those behaviors related to health enhancement, disease prevention, and rehabilitation is called
   a. behavioral health.
   b. psychosomatic medicine.
   c. behavioral medicine.
   d. health psychology.

_____ 17. During the last 25 years of the 20th century, psychology became more involved in people's health mostly by
   a. practicing psychosomatic medicine.
   b. investigating those behaviors that enhance health and prevent disease.
   c. treating mental diseases.
   d. treating physical diseases.

Multiple Choice Answers

1.	a	10.	d
2.	d	11.	c
3.	a	12.	b
4.	a	13.	c
5.	b	14.	d
6.	c	15.	b
7.	c	16.	d
8.	b	17.	b
9.	a		

Behavioral Health, Behavioral Medicine, and Health Psychology

Find a description for each of the following specialty areas and place each under the correct listing on the figure:

Biopsychology—

Cardiology—

Clinical psychology—

Cognitive psychology—

Developmental psychology—

Epidemiology—

Experimental psychology—

Geriatrics—

Health education—

Immunology—

Industrial psychology—

Neuropsychology—

Nutrition—

Oncology—

Pediatrics—

Personality—

Psychopharmacology—

Psychosomatic medicine—

Public health—

Rehabilitation medicine—

Rehabilitation psychology—

Social psychology—

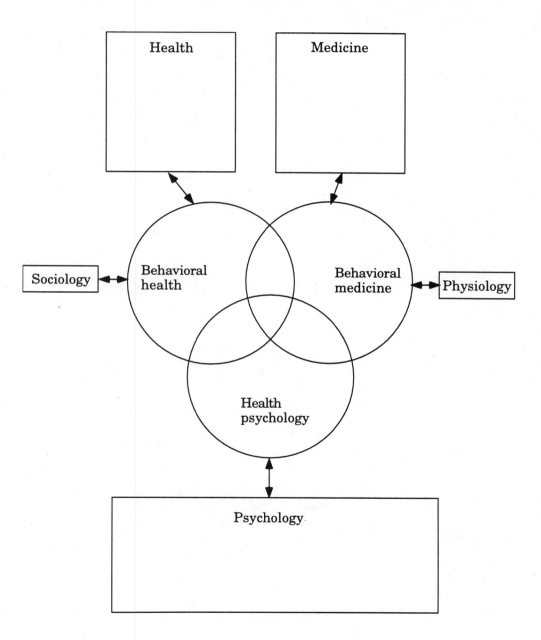

Essay Questions

1.   Discuss the role of ethnicity in health and illness. What factors complicate the interpretation of these effects?

2.   How do behavioral medicine and health psychology differ? How are they similar?

Good points to include in your essay answers:

1.   Ethnicity plays a role in life expectancy.
    A. European Americans have substantially longer life expectancies than African Americans.
    B. The role of ethnicity is not entirely clear because poverty and low socioeconomic status also relate to ethnicity in the United States.
        1. Poverty is related to ethnicity; poor people have restricted access to medical services and lower life expectancy than people with more money.
        2. Low educational level is negatively related to ethnicity, and less educated people are more likely to exhibit risky health-related behaviors.

2.   Behavioral medicine and health psychology have both differences and similarities.
    A. Differences
        1. Behavioral medicine developed as a result of the Yale conference, and health psychology was the result of an APA task force.
        2. Behavioral medicine is an interdisciplinary field; although health psychology has drawn from several fields, it remains within psychology.
        3. The professional societies and journals differ for each area.
        4. The work of those in behavioral medicine tends to concentrate on diagnosis and treatment whereas health psychologists may also be involved in prevention.
    B. Similarities
        1. Both have similar goals, including the integration of biomedical and behavioral knowledge in order to prevent disease and aid in diagnosis and treatment.
        2. Both draw from many fields, including medicine, physiology, psychology, and sociology.
        3. Both health psychologists and those in behavioral medicine can join the others' professional societies and consider the others' journals important to their own work.
        4. The work of health psychologists who concentrate on people who are already ill may be indistinguishable from the work of those in the field of behavioral medicine.

Let's Get Personal—
How Do You Define Health?

What is your personal definition of health—that is, what does being healthy mean? Write down what a healthy person should be and should be able to do. What types of situations or conditions would prevent a person from being healthy?

Does your definition come closer to the biomedical or the biopsychosocial view of health and illness?

What does being healthy mean to you?

A healthy person should be able to:

A person is not healthy if he or she:

Is your view closer to the biomedical or biopsychosocial view?

CHAPTER 2

Conducting Health Research

Fill in the Rest of the Story

I. Scientific Foundations of Health Psychology

Health psychology rests on the foundations of two major disciplines,

psychology and _____. In both disciplines, scientists are

familiar with the work of other scientists, use _____ methods, keep

personal biases from influencing results, make claims cautiously, and

_____ their studies.

II. Contributions of Psychology

Psychology has made five important contributions to health promotion: (1) It

has provided techniques for changing behaviors that relate to _____

disease; (2) It emphasizes _____ rather than disease; (3) It has developed

reliable and _____ instruments for measuring behaviors related to

health; (4) It has created theoretical models to explain and _____

health-related behaviors; and (5) It has used scientific methods for studying

behaviors associated with health and disease.

A. Research Methods in Psychology

Psychologists use a variety of research methods to study human behavior,

including the following: (1) an intensive investigation of one person called a

_____ study; (2) studies that indicate the degree of relationship between two variables, called _____ studies, which are one type of descriptive research; (3) studies conducted at one point in time, called _____-_____ studies; (4) studies that follow participants over an extended period of time, called _____ studies; (5) ex post facto designs, in which the experimenter does not manipulate an _____ variable but selects participants who naturally differ on some subject variable; and (6) experimental designs, in which the investigator manipulates the independent variable and observes its effects on the _____ variable. Experimental designs give scientists their best guess concerning _____; that is, cause and effect. Researchers using an experimental design must control for participants' expectation that treatment will be effective regardless of actual effectiveness. This expectation, which can affect performance, is called the _____ effect. Both psychological and medical placebos provide improvement in about a _____ percent of participants, but these effects can also produce adverse reactions, called the _____ effect.

III. Contributions of Epidemiology

That branch of medicine that investigates factors contributing to the occurrence of a disease in a particular population is called _____. When epidemiologists talk about the proportion of the population affected by a particular disease at a particular time, they use the term

_____, and when they talk about the number of new cases of a

disease during a particular time, they use the term _____.

A. Research Methods in Epidemiology

Research methods in epidemiology are similar to those used in psychology.

Three broad areas of epidemiological study relate to health psychology:

observational methods, natural experiments, and experimental investigations.

Observational methods parallel _____ studies in psychology.

The two types of observational methods are (1) studies that begin with a group of

people already suffering from a disease and are called _____

studies and (2) longitudinal studies that follow the forward development of a

group of people and are called _____ studies.

Retrospective studies are also called _____-_____ studies

because cases (people with a disease) are compared to controls (people not

affected). A group of people starting an experience together is referred to as a

_____. Natural experiments are similar to _____ _____

_____ studies in psychology in that both involve the selection rather

than the manipulation of a variable. Natural experiments can be conducted

when two similar groups of people naturally divide themselves into those exposed

and those not exposed to a pathogen. Experimental investigations are relatively

rare in epidemiology because epidemiologists seldom are in position to

manipulate the _____ variable. The two most common types of

experimental designs are _____ trials and community trials. Experimental designs in epidemiology, just as those in psychology, ordinarily require a _____ - _____ procedure in which neither the participants nor the experimenters directly in contact with the participants know who has received the placebo and who has received the independent variable.

B. Two Examples of Epidemiological Studies

Two examples of these techniques are the classical work of John Snow and the current Alameda County Study. Snow's solution to the London cholera epidemic during the middle of the 19th century was to shut off the supply of polluted _____. The Alameda County Study found that people who practiced six or seven basic health-related behaviors were less likely to die than those who practiced zero to three. These behaviors included (1) getting seven or eight hours of sleep daily, (2) eating breakfast almost every day, (3) rarely eating between meals, (4) drinking alcohol in moderation or not at all, (5) not _____, (6) exercising regularly, and (7) maintaining _____ near the prescribed ideal.

C. Evaluation of Research Methods

Both psychological and epidemiological studies have some weakness. First, most merely indicate a _____ between a behavior and an outcome and do not prove a cause-and-effect relationship. Second, most rely on measuring instruments with limited reliability and _____. Third, many fail to consider the strength of the _____ effect.

IV. Determining Causation

Most epidemiological studies do not prove causation; rather, they point to

specific _____ factors that are associated with a particular disease

or disorder.

A. The Risk Factor Approach

A risk factor is any characteristic or condition that occurs with greater

frequency in people with a disease than it does in people free from that disease.

Although they do not determine causation, risk factors can be used to determine

the _____ of developing a disease. Scientists using the risk

factor approach must distinguish between two kinds of risks: (1)

_____ risk, which is the ratio between the number of people in an

exposed group with a disease and the number in an unexposed group with the

disease; and (2) _____ risk, which refers to a person's chance of

developing a disease independent of the risk for other people.

B. Cigarettes and Disease: Is There a Causal Relationship?

Although scientists have no evidence from _____ designs

proving that cigarette smoking causes heart disease and lung cancer, the

accumulation of other evidence strongly suggest a causal relationship. First, the

more people smoke, the more they are likely to suffer from a disease. This is

called a _____ - _____ response relationship. Second, the

prevalence and incidence of a disease declines when people _____

smoking. Third, cigarette smoking _____ development of disease rather than vice versa. Forth, the relationship between cigarette smoking and disease makes sense from a _____ viewpoint. Fifth, relevant research yields a consistent pattern of results—a pattern that has been established through _____ - _____, a statistical technique that allows the combination of information from several studies into one analysis. Sixth, the size of the relative risk is large—about 2.0 for cardiovascular disease and 9.0 for _____ _____. Seventh, the evidence is based on a number of well-designed studies. A combination of these criteria can allow epidemiologists to determine causality from nonexperimental designs.

V. Research Tools

A. The Role of Theory in Research

Theories are scientific tools that researchers use to determine areas of inquiry and to test hypotheses. A set of related assumptions from which testable hypotheses can be drawn is one definition of a _____. Theories allow researchers to _____ data and render them meaningful, generate descriptive research, suggest a variety of _____ that can be tested, and follow a guideline for working through daily problems.

B. The Role of Psychometrics in Health Psychology

Health psychologists, like other scientists, use measuring instruments to test their hypotheses and build their theories. To be useful, measuring devices must be both _____ (consistent) and _____ (accurate).

Answers

I.   epidemiology; controlled; replicate
II.   chronic; health; valid; predict
II. A.   case; correlational; cross-sectional; longitudinal; independent; dependent; causation; placebo; 35%; nocebo
III.   epidemiology; prevalence; incidence
III. A. correlational; retrospective; prospective; case-control; cohort; ex post facto; independent; clinical; double-blind
III. B. water; smoking; weight
III. C. relationship (correlation); validity; placebo
IV.   risk
IV. A.   probability (risk); relative; absolute
IV. B.   experimental; dose-response; stop (quit); precedes; biological; meta-analysis; lung cancer
V.A.   theory; organize; hypotheses
V.B.   reliable; valid

Multiple Choice Questions

_____   1.   While listening to a morning television program, you hear a TV personality report that he lowered his resting heart rate by 15 beats per minute as a result of self-hypnosis. Such a report
          a.   is good evidence of the effectiveness self-hypnosis in lowering heart rate.
          b.   should be considered a testimonial and given little or no credence.
          c.   should be considered as a case study.
          d.   is an example of an ex post facto study.

_____   2.   A weakness of the case study method is that
          a.   It has no theoretical implications.
          b.   It does not allow generalization.
          c.   It requires several decades to complete.
          d.   It is more costly than multiple-participant designs.

_____   3.   As X increases, so does Y; as X decreases, so does Y. This relationship suggests that X and Y are
          a.   negatively skewed.
          b.   positively skewed.
          c.   positively correlated.
          d.   negatively correlated.

_____ 4. Cancer and heart disease can be investigated by using this method:
   a. experimental design.
   b. ex post facto design.
   c. descriptive research.
   d. all or any of the above

_____ 5 Descriptive studies include
   a. experimental designs.
   b. correlation studies.
   c. both of the above.
   d. neither a nor b

_____ 6. Any condition that occurs with greater frequency in people with a disease than in people free from that disease is known as
   a. a correlational factor.
   b. a placebo effect.
   c. an extraneous variable.
   d. a risk factor.
   e. none of the above

_____ 7. A study that uses participants of at least two different age groups or developmental periods is called a(n)
   a. experimental study.
   b. ex post facto design.
   c. longitudinal study.
   d. cross-sectional study.

_____ 8. An important disadvantage of the longitudinal study is that it
   a. requires a team of researchers.
   b. is time consuming.
   c. is limited to retrospective designs.
   d. is limited to ex post facto designs.

_____ 9. Which of these is the best example of a longitudinal study?
   a. a survey that compares college freshmen with their grandparents on attitudes toward health care
   b. a clinical trial shows that AZT is an effective drug for slowing the rate of HIV infection
   c. a study which finds that level of education is inversely related to death rate from cardiovascular disease
   d. a study that follows the natural history of drug use in female participants over a 20 year period

_____ 10. An investigator measures blood pressure in a group of college seniors and then repeats these measures every year for 20 years. This is an example of
a. a longitudinal study.
b. a cross-sectional study.
c. an experimental study.
d. a clinical trial.

_____ 11. Determining the cause of a disease most accurately depends on
a. single-participant designs.
b. case control studies.
c. correlational studies.
d. experimental designs.

_____ 12. In a study that examines the effects of exercise on coronary heart disease, exercise would be
a. the dependent variable.
b. the independent variable.
c. a placebo effect.
d. an extraneous variable.

_____ 13. An experimental study looks at the effects of stress on heart disease in elderly women. The dependent variable in such a study is
a. gender.
b. age.
c. heart disease.
d. stress.

_____ 14. The expectancy effect is also known as the
a. self-efficacy effect.
b. placebo effect.
c. double-blind effect.
d. epinephrine effect.

_____ 15 To determine if Drug X lowers blood pressure, scientists would administer Drug X to an experimental group and _____ to a comparison group.
a. a placebo
b. Drug Z
c. a lower dose of Drug X
d. a higher dose of Drug X

_____ 16. With regard to the placebo effect, one can most accurately say that it is
  a. physiologically real but not capable of alleviating organic symptoms.
  b. physiologically real and capable of alleviating some organic symptoms.
  c. most likely to be manifested in well-designed experiments.
  d. an imaginary effect and thus not important.

_____ 17. Research designs that are similar to experimental designs but do not include manipulation of the independent variable are called
  a. ex post facto designs.
  b. correlational studies.
  c. cross-sectional studies.
  d. case studies.

_____ 18. That branch of medicine that investigates factors contributing to increased health or the occurrence of a disease in a particular population is called
  a. health psychology.
  b. statistical health analysis.
  c. public health.
  d. epidemiology.

_____ 19. The number of new cases of AIDS in a given year is called
  a. rate of illness.
  b. rate of death.
  c. prevalence.
  d. incidence.

_____ 20. The percentage of the population that has a disease in any one period of time is called
  a. incidence.
  b. prevalence.
  c. correlational evidence.
  d. an epidemic.

_____ 21. Retrospective studies
  a. are a type of correlational studies.
  b. begin with a group of participants who are disease-free and then follow them for a number of years.
  c. begin with a group of participants already suffering from a disease.
  d. are a type of case study.

_____ 22. An epidemiological prospective study would also be
     a. longitudinal.
     b. correlational.
     c. cross-sectional.
     d. none of the above

_____ 23. In a case-control study
     a. people affected by a disease are compared with people not affected by that disease.
     b. one person is studied in detail over a short period of time.
     c. one person is studied on one characteristic over a long period of time.
     d. the responses of one group of people are correlated with the responses of another group.

_____ 24. A person who has a risk factor for cardiovascular disease
     a. will develop cardiovascular disease if he or she lives long enough.
     b. will not develop cardiovascular disease unless he or she has two or more risk factors.
     c. is more likely to develop cardiovascular disease than someone without the risk factor.
     d. exhibits some of the behavioral as well as some of the physical causes for cardiovascular disease.

_____ 25. When people are allowed to decide to be in either the experimental group or the control group, this becomes a serious problem:
     a. the placebo effect.
     b. the ethical treatment of human participants.
     c. the double-blind effect.
     d. self-selection.

_____ 26. Which of these is an example of an epidemiological field study?
     a. an ex post facto study
     b. a community trial
     c. a clinical trial
     d. a case study

_____ 27 Morbidity is to mortality as
     a. illness is to disease.
     b. disease is to death.
     c. death is to disease.
     d. death is to trauma.

_____ 28. You hear on the radio that researchers have found a significant negative correlation between eating tomatoes and developing prostate cancer. From this, you can infer that
   a. eating tomatoes causes lower rates of prostate cancer.
   b. eating tomatoes causes higher rates of prostate cancer.
   c   nothing about cause and effect.
   d. the study was an experimental design.

_____ 29. These studies best determine cause and effect:
   a. cross-sectional.
   b. case studies.
   c. experimental designs.
   d. clinical trials.

_____ 30. One function of a useful theory is to
   a. introduce bias in research.
   b. eliminate bias in research.
   c. generate research.
   d. be proven true.

_____ 31. If a test is reliable it is
   a. valid.
   b. truthful.
   c. consistent.
   d. based on factor analytic data.

Multiple Choice Answers

1.	b		16.	b
2.	b		17.	a
3.	c		18.	d
4.	d		19.	d
5.	b		20.	b
6.	d		21.	c
7.	d		22.	a
8.	b		23.	a
9.	d		24.	c
10.	a		25.	d
11.	d		26.	b
12.	b		27.	b
13.	c		28.	c
14.	b		29.	c
15.	a		30.	c
			31.	c

Match these important authorities to their work:

1. Ray Rosenman

2. John Snow

3. Lisa Berkman and Lester Breslow

4. Sir Francis Galton

a. pioneered the measurement of human abilities.

b. one of the originators of the Type A behavior pattern.

c. developed statistical analysis techniques used in psychology research.

d. conducted the Alameda County study.

e. pioneer epidemiologist.

1. b   2. e   3. d   4. a

Experimental Design—

Can a Low-Fat Diet Lower Cholesterol Level?

Your textbook includes an example of an experimental design that manipulates diet as the independent variable and measures changes in risk factors for cardiovascular disease (CVD). Figure 2.1 shows this design, which will allow researchers to answer the question, "Does changing diet change the level of risk for CVD?"

In the figure that follows, fill in the missing information for an experiment to determine the influence of a low-fat diet on lowering cholesterol level. In this study, the type of diet (low-fat versus regular) is the independent variable, and change in cholesterol level is the dependent variable. Complete the missing information:

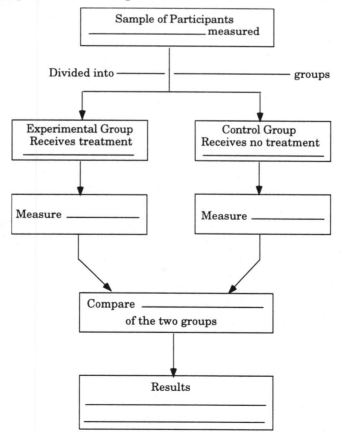

Sample of Participants
_____ measured

Divided into ————— | ————————— groups

Experimental Group
Receives treatment
_____

Control Group
Receives no treatment
_____

Measure _____

Measure _____

Compare _____
of the two groups

Results
_____
_____

Essay Questions

1. What is a placebo and how can it affect research and treatment?

2.   Your instructor tells you to design and conduct a study that would demonstrate that cigarettes cause lung cancer. What would be the barriers to your project? What would you need to do to complete the assignment?

Good points to include in your essay answers:

1.   A placebo is a treatment that is capable of causing effects through expectation of the effectiveness of the treatment, independent of the influence of the treatment itself. It has effects for both research and treatment.
     A.   Placebo effects in research are a problem.
          1.   People expect treatments to work and respond according to their expectancies rather than according to the treatment.
          2.   The response to placebos creates an inflated assessment of the effectiveness of both medical and psychological treatment.
          3.   Researchers must include some control procedures to allow for the accurate assessment of treatment effectiveness.
     B.   Placebo effects are an advantage in treatment situations.
          1.   Placebos bring about improvements and cures that are indistinguishable from those brought about by medically and psychologically effective treatments.
          2.   The placebo effect can add to the effect of medical and psychological treatment, boosting the effectiveness.

2.   To determine causation, the study would have to be an experiment with human participants.
     A.   The experiment should
          1.   Begin with a representative sample of the population.
          2.   Randomly assign participants to two equal groups—smoking and nonsmoking.
               a.   The smoking group would be required to smoke.
               b.   The nonsmoking group would be prohibited from smoking.
          3.   Continue for at least 20 years, with the lives of both groups being equivalent except for smoking.
          4.   Determine cause of death for all participants who died, comparing lung cancer deaths between the two groups.
          5.   Allow conclusions concerning the causal role of smoking in the development of lung cancer.
     B.   The proposed experiment poses several problems.
          1.   Ethical problem result from the smoking requirement; those in the smoking group would not be allowed to decline participation.
          2.   Practical problems would arise as a result of the longitudinal nature of the study and the amount of control over the people during the study.

Let's Get Personal—
Epidemiologists at Work

Your opportunities to be involved in epidemiology research are few, but you can see a dramatization of some very important epidemiology research by seeing *And the Band Played On*, which is available on video. This movie depicts the development of the AIDS epidemic and the search for its cause by the epidemiologists at the Centers for Disease Control and Prevention. In addition to the political complexities, the movie shows the field and laboratory research that identified the human immunodeficiency virus.

How did the CDC initially become aware that some new disease was spreading?

How did epidemiologists identify the modes of transmission for HIV infection?

How did epidemiologists identify the risk factors for HIV infection?

What were the barriers that slowed the identification of the modes of transmission and risk factors?

In addition to epidemiologists, what researchers were involved with understanding AIDS?

CHAPTER 3
Seeking Health Care

Fill in the Rest of the Story

I. Adopting Health-Related Behaviors

Although health is highly valued, people do not always behave in ways that promote their health.

A. Theories of Health-Protective Behaviors

Several theories attempt to explain health-related behaviors. The health belief model includes four factors that should combine to predict health-related behaviors: perceived _____ to disease or disability, perceived _____ of the disease or disability, perceived benefits of health-enhancing behaviors, and perceived _____ to health-enhancing behaviors.

The theory of reasoned action assumes that people are quite reasonable and make systematic use of information when deciding how to behave. According to this theory, the immediate determinant of behavior is a person's _____ to act, which in turn is shaped by one's attitude toward the behavior and one's perception of the social pressure to perform or not perform the action; that is, one's _____ _____.

The theory of planned behavior is an extension of the theory of reasoned

32

action, adding people's perception of their control over behavior. The ease or difficulty of achieving desired behavioral outcomes is called perceived _____ control and reflects both past behaviors and perceived ability to overcome obstacles.

Albert Bandura's social cognitive theory of self-regulation is a general theory of behavior that stresses the interaction of behavior, environment, and person factors, especially cognition, an interaction called _____ _____. An important part of the person factor is one's perceived ability to perform behaviors necessary to bring about a desired consequence, a component called _____ - _____.

Neil Weinstein's _____ adoption process model assumes that when people begin new and relatively complex behaviors aimed at protecting themselves from harm, they go through as many as seven stages of belief about their personal susceptibility. In Stage 1, people are unaware of the hazard. In Stage 2, they are aware of the hazard but believe that, although others are at risk, they are not—a situation Weinstein calls an _____ _____. People in Stage 3 acknowledge their _____ and accept the notion that precaution would be personally effective. Action occurs in Stage 4, whereas in the parallel Stage 5 people decide that action is _____. In Stage 6, people have already taken the precaution aimed at reducing risks, and Stage 7 involves _____ the precaution.

The transtheoretical model of James Prochaska assumes that people progress through five stages in making changes in behavior: _____, contemplation, preparation, action, and maintenance. People in the first stage may fail to see that they have a problem. The stage that involves awareness of the problem and thoughts about changing behavior is _____, but people in this stage have not yet made an effort to change. The stage that includes thoughts, actions, and specific plans about change is called preparation. Modification of behavior comes in the _____ stage when people make overt changes in their behavior. During the _____ stage, people try to sustain the changes they have made and to resist temptation to relapse.

B. Critique of Health-Related Theories

How do these health-related theories meet criteria of a useful theory; that is, how well do they (1) generate _____, (2) organize and _____ observations, and (3) help the practitioner predict and change behaviors? None of the models are able to completely explain the complexities of health-related behavior, but the concepts of intention and self-_____ have supporting research.

II. Seeking Medical Attention

How people determine their health status when they don't feel well depends on their social and cultural background, their interpretation of symptoms, and their concept of what constitutes illness. Those activities by people who feel sick, and that are directed toward determining health status before an official

diagnosis, are called _____ behaviors, whereas those activities

exhibited by people after they have been diagnosed, and that are aimed at trying

to get well, are _____ _____ behaviors.

A. Illness Behavior

Many people have a personal reluctance to seek medical care. They are

willing to advise others to see a doctor, but with the same symptoms, they are

_____ to go to the doctor themselves. Several social and

demographic factors predict willingness to seek professional care. One is gender,

and _____ are more likely than _____ to seek health

care. Socioeconomic level is another factor; people at the upper levels are less

likely than those at the lower levels to become sick, but they are

_____ likely to seek health care and to do so more quickly when

they become ill. Young and middle-aged people show more reluctance to seek

health care than older adults. Stress is also a factor in seeking health care, with

stress _____ the likelihood of seeking health care.

Symptom characteristics also influence how people respond to illness.

People are most likely to seek medical care when their symptoms are visible to

themselves and to others, when they view the symptoms as

_____, when their symptoms interfere with their usual

_____, and when their symptoms recur or _____.

People's personal view of illness depends both on their knowledge of the illness and on their previously formed cognitions. Young children often believe that illness occurs for no apparent reason or because of "_____." Additional cognitive development is needed to grasp the notion that personal _____ can affect health. Still greater cognitive development is necessary before people can understand that psychological, social, and physiological factors interact to cause illness.

Howard Leventhal and his colleagues identified four components in the conceptualization of illness. First is the identity of the disease.   People need to label their symptoms, and such a label seems to alleviate symptom anxieties. Second, the _____ _____ helps people conceptualize illness. When people receive a diagnosis, they think about the time course of both the disease and the treatment. Third, people think of the consequences of their disease, and fourth they attribute a _____ to their symptoms.

B. The Sick Role

After people become convinced that they are ill, they adopt the _____ _____. One premise of the sick role is that sick people are not to blame for their illness, but research has shown that lack of _____ may not be an accurate description of the sick role. Sick people are usually exempt from attending school, going to work, cooking meals, or cleaning house. Their obligations include acting sick while also being optimistic, cheerful, and brave, which may add more stress to being ill.

C. Choosing a Practitioner

Part of seeking health care is choosing a practitioner—a physician or one of the many alternative types of health care practitioners. As medicine has become more complex, technological, and corporate, patients have adopted a consumer attitude toward medicine. Nearly one-third now choose "_____" health care. Young patients, especially, are likely to _____ the authority of physicians.

III. Being in the Hospital

Being in the hospital can be a stressful experience for several reasons. In addition to being sick, hospitalized patients must cope with the hospital routine and deal with the possibility of distressing medical procedures.

A. The Hospital Patient Role

Being a patient means conforming to rules of the health care institution and complying with medical advice. Many hospitalized patients become almost invisible to the hospital staff and are treated as though they were not present; that is, they receive _____ treatment. Well-informed patients tend to be less stressed than poorly informed ones, but traditionally, hospitalized patients have experienced a _____ of information about their condition. Patients who must conform to hospital routine and are not allowed to make the everyday decisions experience a loss of _____, which often adds more stress to an already stressful situation.

B. "Good" Patients Versus "Bad" Patients

Most patients conform to hospital routine and are considered "good" patients, but a significant number complain, ask questions, demand answers, and are regarded as _____ patients. When patients react angrily in an attempt to restore control, these angry behaviors are called

_____. Being a bad patient may be healthier than being a good patient because good patients may accept their illness and feel helpless.

Feelings of learned _____ can lead to passivity and sometimes to depression.

IV. Preparing for Stressful Medical Procedures

Hospitalization can include the added worry of stressful medical procedures. Psychologists have identified two different styles of coping with stressful medical procedures, people who become overly vigilant and anxious and are called

_____ and people who tend to ignore and deny problems, the

_____.

A. Techniques for Coping

In reducing anxiety in patients facing stressful medical treatment, information about procedures that will be used is generally less effective than information about _____ that patients will experience. Relaxation techniques are generally successful in reducing the stress associated with medical procedures but may not be sufficient for serious procedures. Learning by watching others perform, which psychologists call

_____, has also been used to help patients cope with stressful medical procedures, especially when the model is initially seen as being anxious and then overcoming the anxiety.

B. Children and Hospitalization

Children are especially vulnerable to persistent fears as a result of receiving medical treatment. One effective strategy with children includes allowing them to express their emotions by playing with _____. Trust in the medical staff can be built through films, hospital tours, books, and by permitting parents to stay with the child. Children also profit from the same techniques used with adults, namely relaxation training, peer models, distraction, and self-talk.

Answers

I.A. susceptibility; severity; barriers; intention; subjective norm; behavioral; eciprocal determinism; self-efficacy; precaution; optimistic bias; risk; (susceptibility); unnecessary; maintaining; precontemplation; contemplation; action; maintenance

I.B. research; explain; efficacy

II. illness; sick role

II.A. reluctant (unwilling); women; men; more; increasing; severe (serious); lifestyle (activities or routine); persist; magic; behavior (actios); time line; cause (reason)

II.B. sick role; blame

II.C. alternative; challenge.

III.A nonperson; lack; control

III.B. bad; reactance; helplessness

IV. Sensitizers; Repressors

IV.A sensations; modeling

IV.B. puppets (toys)

Multiple Choice Questions

_____ 1. Psychologists use theories to
a. predict behavior.
b. explain behavior.
c. both a and b
d. neither a nor b

_____ 2. The theory that includes the concepts of perceived susceptibility to disease, perceived severity of the disease, perceived benefits of health-enhancing behaviors, and perceived barriers to health-enhancing behaviors is
a. the theory of planned behavior.
b. the theory of reasoned action.
c. the precaution adoption process model.
d. the health belief model.

_____ 3. Although _____ has produced the most extensive research on health-related behaviors, research testing its usefulness has been somewhat inconsistent.
a. the health belief model
b. the theory of planned behavior
c. the adoption precaution process model
d. the transtheoretical model

_____ 4. This theory assumes that the immediate cause of people's actions are their intentions to act.
a. the health belief model
b. the transtheoretical model
c. the precaution adoption process model
d. the theory of reasoned action

_____ 5. According to the theory of reasoned action, a person's perception of the social pressure to perform or not perform an action is called
a. perceived severity of one's illness.
b. subjective norm.
c. attitude toward the behavior.
d. optimistic bias.

_____ 6. Which of these concepts is crucial to the theory of reasoned action?
a. internal locus of control
b. perceived severity of the disease
c. intention to act
d. perceived susceptibility to a disease

_____ 7. Perceived behavioral control is a key concept in this theory:
  a. transtheoretical model
  b. behavior modification
  c. theory of reasoned action
  d. theory of planned behavior

_____ 8. A key element in Albert Bandura's self-regulation theory is
  a. subjective norms.
  b. intention to behave.
  c. self-efficacy.
  d. internal locus of control.

_____ 9. According to Albert Bandura's idea of reciprocal determinism, human conduct is influenced by
  a. behavior.
  b. environment.
  c. person factors.
  d. an interaction among a, b, and c

_____ 10. People's beliefs that they can perform those behaviors necessary to bring about control over events that affect their lives is called
  a. external locus of control.
  b. overconfidence.
  c. self-efficacy.
  d. outcome expectancy.

_____ 11. Neil Weinstein suggested that, when people begin new and relatively complex behaviors aimed at protecting themselves from harm, they go through a series of beliefs about their personal susceptibility. This model of behavior is called the
  a. the transtheoretical model.
  b. theory of planned behavior.
  c. self-regulation theory.
  d. the precaution adoption process model.

_____ 12. Dallas, like most of his friends, does not exercise regularly. He believes that his sedentary friends are susceptible to heart disease, but he exempts himself from any high risk. Weinstein would say that Dallas
  a. will take action to protect himself.
  b. is in Stage 6 of the adoption precaution process.
  c. has an optimistic bias.
  d. will eventually develop heart disease.

_____ 13. Precontemplation, contemplation, preparation, action, and maintenance are five concepts central to this theory.
   a. self-regulation
   b. transtheoretical model
   c. adoption precaution process model
   d. theory of reasoned action

_____ 14. Which of these is a reason that theories fail to predict health-related behavior?
   a. The theories are not based on psychological constructs.
   b. Health-seeking behavior is sometimes limited by poverty and public policy.
   c. The theories are applied too specifically to health-related behavior.
   d. The theories are psychological and not medical.

_____ 15. After feeling ill for 2 days, Angelo went to his doctor who diagnosed his illness as influenza and prescribed bed rest and medication. Angelo had the prescription filled, took the medication, and went to bed. Angelo's behavior after seeing his doctor would be considered
   a. illness behavior.
   b. sick role behavior.
   c. reluctance behavior.
   d. reactance behavior.

_____ 16. People's actions designed to determine their health status are called
   a. sick role behaviors.
   b. illness behaviors.
   c. health-seeking behaviors.
   d. premature diagnoses.

_____ 17. Research on personal reluctance suggests that if both Kyle and Cameron are experiencing the same symptoms, Kyle is likely to
   a. advise Cameron to seek health care but not to do so himself.
   b. convince both himself and Cameron not to seek health care.
   c. seek health care but advise Cameron not to.
   d. see his symptoms as more serious than Cameron's.

_____ 18. In general, who is MOST likely to seek medical care?
   a. women
   b. men
   c. low income people
   d. Irish Americans

_____ 19. Howard Leventhal and his associates consider _____ to be a component in people's conceptualization of illness.
- a. the monetary cost of treatment
- b. the consequence of the illness
- c. the competence level of the physician
- d. all of the above

_____ 20. Morgan has not been feeling well lately. In trying to diagnose himself, Morgan is likely to
- a. deny the existence of his symptoms.
- b. try to find a nonthreatening label that fits his symptoms.
- c. exaggerate his symptoms so as to imagine the most serious consequences.
- d. repress his symptoms.

_____ 21. As part of the sick role, Talcott Parsons contended that
- a. labeling symptoms makes people feel more anxious.
- b. labeling symptoms makes people feel less anxious.
- c. being sick adds to the person's normal responsibilities.
- d. being sick is not the sick person's fault.

_____ 22. Richard Lazarus contended that sick people often have added stress in their life because
- a. they are usually expected to be cheerful, brave, and optimistic.
- b. they are frequently expected to be depressed, pessimistic, and frightened.
- c. they must accept responsibility for their illness as well as for their treatment.
- d. other people have a tendency to avoid them.

_____ 23. Patients are most likely to be satisfied with physicians who
- a. keep current with the latest technology.
- b. have a high level of knowledge and skill.
- c. act through power and authority.
- d. are caring, communicative, and reassuring.
- e. are professional and reserved in their demeanor.

_____ 24. From the point of view of the hospital staff, the ideal patient would be
- a. very intelligent.
- b. very talkative.
- c. unconscious.
- d. dead.
- e. robot-like.

_____ 25. To fulfill the "good patient" role, a hospitalized patient should
   a. become involved as a cooperative partner in the health care he or she receives.
   b. become capable of making independent decisions about his or her care.
   c. be obedient and avoid questioning hospital routine.
   d. occasionally become angry, venting negative feelings and frustrations.

_____ 26. Hospitalized people who are "bad patients"
   a. become unresponsive unless a hospital staff member speaks to them.
   b. become angry and fail to comply with hospital routine.
   c. appear similar to "good patients" but experience difference emotions.
   d. become depressed.

_____ 27. People who are described by the label _____ do better   when they receive information about the medical procedures they are undergoing, whereas _____ do better when they do not receive information.
   a. active copers . . . avoidant copers
   b. reactant copers . . . relevant copers
   c. avoidant copers . . . assimilant copers
   d. resistant copers . . . reactive copers

_____ 28. The effectiveness of relaxation as a technique for coping with stressful medical procedures is best described as
   a. very successful with all medical procedures.
   b. successful with major medical procedures, but not with minor ones.
   c. successful with minor medical procedures, but not with major ones.
   d. not at all successful.

_____ 29. Tomorrow morning Candice's daughter Laura is scheduled for surgery to remove a benign tumor. Because Laura is anxious about the surgery, Candice reassures her by saying, "Everything willturn out fine. You have nothing to worry about." These words are likely to
   a. increase Laura's fear and anxiety.
   b. decrease Laura's anxiety but increase her fear.
   c. decrease Laura's fear and anxiety.
   d. allow Laura to sleep well tonight.

Multiple Choice Answers

1.	c	16.	b
2	d	17.	a
3.	a	18.	a
4.	d	19.	b
5.	b	20.	b
6.	c	21.	d
7.	d	22.	a
8.	c	23.	d
9.	d	24.	e
10.	c	25.	c
11.	d	26.	b
12.	c	27.	a
13.	b	28.	c
14.	b	29.	a
15.	b		

Match the researchers to their research:

1. Neil Weinstein

2. Talcott Parsons

3. Albert Bandura

4. David Mechanic

5. Geoffrey Hochbaum and his colleagues

6. James Prochaska and his colleagues

7. Judith Lorber

8. Icek Ajzen and Martin Fishbein

9. Icek Ajzen

10. Martin Seligman

a. developed the health belief model.

b. studied symptom characteristics and their relation to seeking health care.

c. distinguished between "good patients" and "bad patients."

d. developed the concept of learned helplessness.

e. formulated the concept of self-efficacy, which is the basis for self-regulation theory.

f. developed the precaution adoption process model.

g. developed the theory of reasoned action.

h. developed the transtheoretical model.

i. extended the theory of reasoned action, creating the theory of planned behavior.

j. described the components of the sick role.

1. f   2. j   3. e   4. b   5. a   6. h   7. c
8. g   9. i   10. d

Theory of Reasoned Action in Action

Austin has been thinking about beginning an exercise program to attain a higher level of physical fitness. He has always thought that running or jogging is the best exercise, but his friend Tyler tells him that weightlifting is an excellent exercise. Not only does weight training lead to better fitness, but it also helps in building upper body strength and improves appearance. Austin considers the advantages of weightlifting and concludes that he would like that type of exercise better than jogging. He wonders about the availability of weightlifting equipment and visits the college gym to examine their equipment. The next time he sees Tyler, Austin tells him that he is considering weight training, and Tyler invites Austin to come to the gym with him the next day. Austin agrees, and they meet at the gym the next day.

Fill in each of the boxes in the figure to match Austin's adoption of an exercise program to the theory of reasoned action:

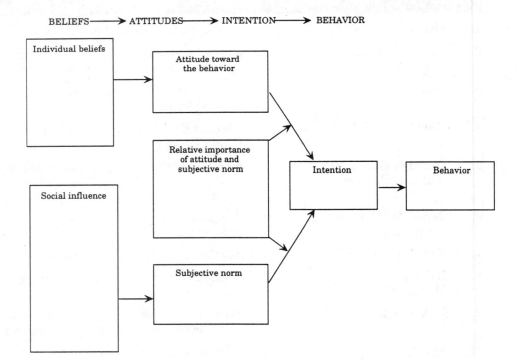

BELIEFS⟶ ATTITUDES ⟶ INTENTION⟶ BEHAVIOR

Individual beliefs

Attitude toward the behavior

Relative importance of attitude and subjective norm

Social influence

Intention

Behavior

Subjective norm

Essay Questions

1. What role do the theories of health-protective behavior serve? How successful are these theories?

2.   Is it better to be a "good" or a "bad" hospital patient?

Good points to include in your essay answers:

1. A. Like all theories, these should
       1. Generate research.
       2. Organize and explain behavior.
       3. Help practitioners change behavior.
    B. The health belief model, theory of reasoned action, theory of planned behavior, self-regulation theory, the precaution adoption model, and the transtheoretical model have been only modestly successful in predicting health-related behaviors.
       1. The health belief model, theory of reasoned action, and self-regulation theory have generated quite a bit of research, but the support for these models has been no better than modest.
       2. All these theories organize and explain behavior, but only some components of the models have been confirmed.
       3. The theories are better at predicting health-seeking behavior than are demographic factors, but all of them leave a great deal unexplained.
       4. With only partial support for any model and failure to explain many facets of health-seeking behavior, practical advice is difficult to formulate.

2. A. "Good" patients
       1. Are obedient, complying with all requests from the hospital staff.
       2. Assume the nonperson role; accept being ignored and helpless.
       3. Conform to hospital routine and do not make extra demands on the hospital staff.
       4. Appear cheerful, regardless of anxiety, fear, pain, or uncertainty.
       5. Do not complain or question anything.
       6. Advantages of the "good patient" role include more attention from the hospital staff, but disadvantages include the possibility of feelings of helplessness and depression.
    B. "Bad" patients
       1. Are disobedient, failing to comply with requests from the hospital staff or some elements of their treatment recommendations.
       2. Do not assume the nonperson role, demand information about their condition, and seek information from the hospital staff.
       3. Fail to conform to all elements of the hospital routine, although these violations are often petty.
       4. Do not appear cheerful and exhibit their anxiety and fear.
       5. Complain.
       6. Disadvantages include the displeasure of the hospital staff but possibly the advantage of conferring feelings of control, which can be an advantage in recovery.

Let's Get Personal—
What Is Sick?

Your personal view of illness affects your behavior when you believe that you are ill. That personal view depends on your knowledge about various diseases and your cognitions about illness. As various researchers have discovered, people who have a sophisticated knowledge about illness may still hold some irrational cognitions about illness.

To explore your illness beliefs, write a description of the last time you were sick. Choose an illness episode that was sufficiently severe to affect your daily routine and cause you to label yourself as sick.

Answer the following questions:

When was the last time you were sick?

What caused you to be sick?

What led you initially to believe that you were sick?

What were the symptoms you noticed?

Was there a time period during which you were not sure that you were sick? If so, what convinced you that you were ill?

Did you receive a diagnosis from a health care professional, or did you diagnose yourself?

How long were you sick?

What changes did you make in your daily activities because you were sick?

What was involved in getting well?

Did you exhibit the typical reluctance to seek medical care by avoiding contact with the medical profession, or did you go to the doctor when you initially experienced symptoms? In either case, what beliefs account for your behavior?

Research indicates that people label their symptoms so that they understand the identity of their illness and that this label is important in understanding the time course and severity of their illness. Is this research consistent with your experience?

When you described what caused you to be sick, did that explanation include a high level of biomedical knowledge? Research indicates that even students with a high level of biological knowledge tend to omit such detail and rely on behavioral factors to explain their illnesses. Is this research consistent with your experience?

CHAPTER 4
Adhering to Medical Advice

Fill In the Rest of the Story

I. The Importance of Adherence

Because the term *compliance* connotes reluctant obedience, many

psychologists prefer _____, cooperation, or collaboration.

II. Theories of Adherence

Several theoretical models that apply to behavior in general have also been

applied to the problem of adherence and nonadherence, including the behavioral

model and several _____ learning theories.

A. The Behavioral Model

The behavioral model is based on the assumption that reinforcers

strengthen behavior, whereas _____ inhibits or suppresses

behavior. Advocates of the behavioral model use cues, _____, and

contracts to reinforce compliant behaviors.

B. Cognitive Learning Theories

Cognitive learning theories extend the concepts of the behavioral model to

include people's interpretation and evaluation of their situation, their emotional

response, and their perceived ability to _____ with illness symptoms.

Self-efficacy refers to people's _____ that they can perform

necessary behaviors to control events that affect their lives. The theory of

_____ action assumes that intentions are the immediate

determinants of behavior and that intention is influenced by

_____ toward the behavior, _____ norms,

and the motivation to comply with these norms.

The _____ _____ model hypothesizes that

four belief states have a cumulative effect for either increasing or decreasing

compliant behavior. These beliefs are (1) perceived _____ to the

negative consequences of nonadherence, (2) perceived severity of these

consequences, (3) the perceived _____/_____ ratio of

performing compliant behaviors, and (4) the perceived _____ to

incorporating adherence behaviors into one's life style.

III. Assessing Adherence

At least five methods have been used to assess patient compliance: (1) ask

the clinician, (2) ask the _____, (3) ask other people, (4) count pills,

and (5) examine biochemical evidence. All approaches have limitations, but the

least valid method is to ask the _____ about rate of patient

compliance.

IV. How Frequent Is Nonadherence?

In general terms, the rate of noncompliance to medical or health advice is

about _____ percent, but about _____ percent of the people who quit

smoking, stop abusing alcohol, or begin an exercise program will eventually

relapse.

V. What Factors Predict Adherence?

Three possible predictors of adherence are (1) illness characteristics,

(2) _____ characteristics, and (3) the practitioner-patient

interaction.

A. Illness Characteristics

Several illness characteristics relate to compliance, but

_____ of the illness as judged by the physician is NOT one of

them. However, severity of the illness as viewed by the _____ does

make some difference. Unpleasant side effects of the treatment are a very

_____ predictor of rate of adherence. Noncompliance tends to

increase as duration of therapy _____. In general, the

greater the variety of medications a person must take, the _____

the likelihood of nonadherence.

B. Personal Characteristics

Personal characteristics such as age, gender, social support, personality

traits, and personal beliefs about health have a complex relationship with patient

compliance. Younger people are usually _____ adherers than

older people. Few overall differences exist in compliance rates for women and

men, but _____ are more likely to adhere to a healthy diet.

Social support is also related to compliance, with married patients

_____ likely to be compliant than those who are not married.

In general, personality traits are a _____ predictor of compliance. Of the various personality variables investigated, two traits emerged as predictors of adherence. In general, obsessive-compulsive people tend to have _____ rates of adherence, whereas _____ individuals tend to have low rates of adherence. Some people cope with illness by denying personal vulnerability. They may smoke more, overeat, or abuse alcohol, strategies called _____ coping. People who believe that they are personally responsible for their own health are _____ likely to be compliant. The relationship between patient and practitioner is a relatively _____ indicator of patient adherence.

C. The Practitioner-Patient Interaction

Perhaps the best predictor of patient compliance is the quality of _____ between practitioner and patient. Patients either fail to remember or misunderstand about _____ percent of the information they receive. Health care professionals are more likely to give advice about diseases than about _____ that maintain or promote health. Patients' compliance improves as confidence in their physician's technical ability _____.

VI. Problems of Adherence

Adherence to medical advice is difficult to predict, even though several factors relate to adherence.

A. Why Are Some People Nonadherent?

Adherence rates are low for at least four reasons. First, adherence broadly defined demands difficult _____ changes, such as changing one's diet, quitting smoking, or beginning an exercise program. Second, many people fail to follow their doctor's advice because they do not correctly hear or

_____ that advice, they stop taking medication when symptoms

_____, or they stop because the symptoms do not seem to

_____. Third, many patients have an _____ bias and

believe that they will be spared the serious consequences of nonadherence.

Fourth, some patients are noncompliant because they have difficulty reading

_____ labels.

B. How Can Adherence Be Improved?

Procedures that impart information boost knowledge but do not usually

result in increased compliance are called _____ strategies.

Behavioral strategies have generally been found to be _____

effective than educational procedures in enhancing patient adherence.

Procedures that increase patient adherence include clearly

_____ instructions, simple prescriptions, _____

- _____ calls for missed appointment, prescriptions tailored to

patient's daily schedule, rewards for compliant behavior, _____ to

signal time for medication, and involving the patient's spouse or social support

network.

C. Does Adherence Pay Off?

In general, research on the health outcomes of adherence are

_____; that is, some studies have shown that people who comply have

better health than those who do not, but other studies have revealed no

_____ between compliance and health.

Answers

I.   adherence
II.   cognitive
II.A.   punishment (punishers); rewards (reinforcers)
II.B.   cope; confidence (belief); reasoned; attitudes; subjective; health belief; susceptibility; cost/benefits; barriers
III.   patient; clinician (physician)
IV.   50; 67
V.   personal (patient)
V.A.   severity; patient; weak; increases; greater (more)
V.B.   worse (poorer); women; more; weak (poor); higher; hostile; avoidance; more; strong (good)
V.C.   communication; 50; behaviors; increases
VI.A.   lifestyle; understand; disappear; improve (go away); optimistic; prescription (medication or drug)
VI.B.   educational; more; written; follow-up; cues (prompts)
VI.C.   inconsistent (unclear); relationship

Multiple Choice Questions

_____ 1. Health psychologists often avoid the term *compliance* because it connotes
  a. cooperation.
  b. defiance.
  c. meekly yielding to outside pressure.
  d. defiantly yielding to outside pressure.

_____ 2. Health psychologists suggest that the ideal relationship between patient and physician should be one of
  a. cooperation.
  b. compliance.
  c. obedience.
  d. reactance.

_____ 3. According to the broad definition of compliance discussed in your textbook, the following behavior would be regarded as compliant:
  a. smoking cigarettes.
  b. continuing to take medication as prescribed even after one's symptoms have disappeared.
  c. discontinuing medication when the symptoms disappear.
  d. failing to keeping an appointment with an oncologist for fear of being diagnosed with cancer.

_____ 4. The behavioral model of adherence
   a. includes the concept of subjective norms.
   b. is less effective than support groups in reducing friction in families with adolescent diabetics.
   c. emphasizes punishment of noncompliant behaviors.
   d. emphasizes reinforcement of compliant behaviors.

_____ 5. This model of compliance emphasizes rewards for compliant behaviors:
   a. the theory of reasoned action
   b. the behavioral model
   c. the adoption precaution process model
   d. the transtheoretical model

_____ 6. Adolescent diabetics frequently fail to comply to their regimen. Research with behavioral strategies reveals that these programs
   a. are more effective than support groups.
   b. are more effective with adolescents 16 to 19 than with adolescents 13 to 15.
   c. are less effective than those that follow the theory of reasoned action.
   d. are ineffective.

_____ 7. Perceived susceptibility, perceived severity, perceived costs/benefits ratio, and perceived barriers are four components of
   a. the health belief model.
   b. self-efficacy theory.
   c. the theory of reasoned action.
   d. the transtheoretical model

_____ 8. Research suggests that physicians tend to
   a. accurately estimate rate of patient compliance.
   b. underestimate rate of patient compliance.
   c. overestimate rate of patient compliance.
   d. be disinterested in rate of patient compliance.

_____ 9. When patients are asked to rate their own percentage of compliance, they are likely to
   a. overrate their own levels of compliance.
   b. underrate their own levels of compliance
   c. accurately rate their own levels of compliance.
   d. not comprehend the question.

_____ 10. When hospital personnel are asked to monitor and rate patients' level
of compliance,
a. compliance rates often increase.
b. an artificial situation exists that makes accurate assessment of
compliance rates difficult.
c. both a and b
d. neither a nor b

_____ 11. A major difficulty of counting pills to measure compliance is that
a. someone may not count unused pills accurately.
b. the method is less reliable than physician judgment.
c. the missing pills may not have been taken according to directions.
d. seriously ill patients may not be motivated to count pills.

_____ 12. An improvement over the pill count method of assessing compliance is
a. the pill cap microprocessor.
b. judgments of physicians.
c. patients' judgments.
d. examination of empty containers.

_____ 13. An advantage of examining biochemical evidence as a measure of
adherence is that such evidence provides
a. an extremely reliable estimate of adherence.
b. a very valid estimate of adherence.
c. a procedure for assessing outcome.
d. an inexpensive means of assessing adherence.

_____ 14. In general terms, methods of assessing patient compliance
a. are quite reliable.
b. are quite valid.
c. are both reliable and valid.
d. have problems with reliability and validity.

_____ 15. Rates of compliance differ according to a variety of factors, but
generally these rates are about
a. 50%.
b. 75%.
c. 90%.
d. 95%.

_____ 16. In general, the highest rates for compliance occur when
    a. the medication is inexpensive.
    b. the medication is for prevention.
    c. the medication is for curing a disease.
    d. patients have no visible symptoms.

_____ 17. Although characteristics of a disease are not a very valid predictor of compliance, this disease characteristic is more predictive of compliance than other disease characteristics:
    a. a chronic rather than an acute disease.
    b. severity of the disease as seen by the doctor.
    c. severity of the medication's side effects.
    d. severity of the disease as seen by the patient.

_____ 18. Research with health care providers indicated that their compliance rates are
    a. about like those of other people.
    b. much higher than those of other people.
    c. much lower than those of other people.
    d. much lower for lower for medication but higher for diet.

_____ 19. According to the parallel response model, people motivated by Fear Control, compared with those motivated by Danger Control are more likely
    a. to use alcohol or drugs to escape fear of illness.
    b. to experience fear when first learning of severe physical symptoms.
    c. to seek medical care when symptoms first occur.
    d. to behave adaptively in order to control their fear.

_____ 20. Kevin takes prescribed medication infrequently. Kevin's illness probably
    a. has not yet been diagnosed.
    b. is not very painful.
    c. is not a chronic disease.
    d. is not a hereditary disorder.

_____ 21. With regard to noncompliance, which of these statements most clearly agrees with research?
    a. Unpleasant side effects of the treatment are strongly associated with dropping out of a treatment regimen.
    b. The longer people must submit to treatment, the greater the likelihood that they will be noncompliant.
    c. People suffering from a chronic illness are more likely to be compliant than those suffering from an acute illness.
    d. People with no visible symptoms are more likely to be noncompliant than people with obvious symptoms.

_____ 22. Which of these personal factors best predicts compliance?
   a. age
   b. ethnic background
   c. gender
   d. personal beliefs

_____ 23. Whenever Gordon experiences symptoms of angina, he responds by having a few strong drinks of Scotch. Gordon's behavior can best be described as
   a. reasoned action.
   b. avoidance coping.
   c. anger control.
   d. danger control.

_____ 24. Research on the link between personality traits and compliance rates has shown
   a. that obsessive-compulsive people have the highest rates of compliance.
   b. that cynically hostile men have the highest rates of compliance.
   c. that cynically hostile women have the highest rates of compliance.
   d. no relationship between any personality trait and compliance

_____ 25. The following approach is generally LEAST effective in improving compliance rates:
   a. educational messages
   b. cues
   c. rewards
   d. cognitive-behavioral strategies

_____ 26. The relationship between compliance and improved health is
   a. positive.
   b. negative.
   c. curvilinear.
   d. not apparent.

_____ 27. The following approach is generally MOST effective in improving compliance rates:
   a. verbal punishments
   b. educational messages
   c. simple, clearly written instructions
   d. rational explanations concerning the dire consequences of noncompliance

Multiple Choice Answers

1.	c	15.	a
2.	a	16.	c
3.	b	17.	d
4.	d	18.	a
5.	b	19.	a
6.	a	20.	b
7.	a	21.	b
8.	c	22.	d
9.	a	23.	b
10.	c	24.	a
11.	c	25.	a
12.	a	26.	d
13.	c	27.	c
14.	d		

Essay Questions

1. What illness characteristics are related to compliance, and what ones show little relationship?

2. Which is more important in compliance—the person's personality or the person's social circumstances?

Good points to include in your essay answers:

1. A. Patients' perception of illness severity is more important in compliance than physicians' perception of the severity.
    B. Treatments that produce unpleasant side effects result in lower adherence, but side effects are not a major factor in compliance.
    C. Lengthy treatments produce lower adherence than shorter term treatments.
    D. Complex regimens lower compliance.

2. A. Personality traits are not good predictors of compliance.
    1. The noncompliant personality does not exist.
    2. People who are obsessive-compulsive are more compliant, and those who are high in cynical hostility are less compliant.
    B. Personal beliefs in responsibility for health and social circumstances show some relationship to compliance.
    1. Social support for adherence increases compliance.
    2. People whose cultural norms are consistent with the treatment tend to have higher compliance than those with different cultural values.

Let's Get Personal—
What's Your Problem with Compliance?

Unless you are exceptional, you fail to comply with some aspect of exemplary health behavior. Perhaps you have a medicine cabinet full of bottles with only a few pills, indicating that you have failed to take your medication as prescribed. Perhaps you have not had a physical examination in years. Perhaps you eat a high-fat diet, smoke, or fail to exercise regularly. Almost everyone deviates from medical orders in some respect.

Sometimes the problem is knowledge and the failure to understand what is required to follow medical advice. More often, some situational barriers prevent people from doing what they know they should do. Choose a noncompliant behavior and analyze the barriers that prevent you from taking the proper action by answering the following questions:

What is your area of noncompliance?

Do you see this problems as serious?

What are the immediate consequences of your noncompliance?

What are the long-term consequences of your noncompliance?

How likely is it that these consequences will happen to you as opposed to other people who are similarly noncompliant?

What would you need to do to be compliant?

Is this regimen complex, or does it require you to make major changes in your daily routine?

In what ways will your adherence improve your health?

Do your family and friends think that it is important for you to comply with this regimen?

Does anyone remind you of your treatment and help you to adhere to it, or do those around you ignore or even discourage you?

How do you feel about the health care professional who recommended this treatment?

What role do these feelings play in your noncompliance?

How has this health care professional helped you to follow his or her recommendations? Has anything he or she has done discouraged you?

Do you feel that you are an active participant in your health care, or do you feel that you are following orders?

What could motivate you to be more compliant?

CHAPTER 5
Defining and Measuring Stress

Fill in the Rest of the Story

I. The Nervous System and the Physiology of Stress

The nervous system is composed of nerve cells called _____

that provide internal communication by releasing chemical

_____ that flow across the space between neurons called the

_____ cleft. Sensory neurons are also called _____

neurons and transmit information from the sense organs toward the brain,

whereas motor neurons, also called _____ neurons, activate

muscles and glands. The neurons that connect the two are called

_____. The nervous system is divided into two parts; the

_____ _____ system consists of the brain and spinal

cord, and all the other nerves in the body are in the _____

nervous system.

A. The Peripheral Nervous System

The peripheral nervous system is also divided into two divisions, the

_____ nervous system, which activates voluntary muscles, and

the _____ nervous system, which serves internal organs and

glands. The autonomic nervous system (ANS) is divided into the

_____ and _____ divisions. The two

main neurotransmitters of the ANS are acetylcholine and

_____.

B. The Neuroendocrine System

The endocrine system consists of ductless glands, and the

_____ system consists of endocrine glands controlled by the

nervous system. These glands release _____ that travel through

the blood and act on target organs. The _____ gland is located in

the brain and releases a number of hormones that affect target organs in many

parts of the body, including _____ hormone (ACTH), which

acts on the adrenal glands. The _____ glands are located on top

of the kidneys and contain two structures that produce different hormones, the

_____ (outer covering) and the _____ (inner

structure). The adrenal cortex secretes three types of hormones, including

glucocorticoids, the most important of which is _____. The

adrenal medulla is activated by the sympathetic nervous system and secretes

catecholamines, including _____ and

_____.

C. Physiology of the Stress Response

The stress reaction mobilizes body resources in emergency situations by

activating the _____ nervous system and the

_____ system. The pituitary stimulates the adrenal cortex to produce _____, including cortisol. Autonomic processes increase or decrease to meet the demands of the emergency situation. The action occurs as a result of the secretion of two adrenal hormones, _____. and _____.

II. Theories of Stress

Hans Selye and Richard Lazarus have proposed influential theories of stress.

A. Selye's View

Selye's theory defined stress as a generalized or _____ response to a variety of environmental stressors. Selye hypothesized that the response to stress occur in three stages, which taken together, are called the

_____ _____ _____.

These three stages are _____, followed by resistance, and then _____. A criticism of Selye's theory is that it concentrates on the physiological and downplays the _____ aspects of stress.

B. Lazarus's View

To Lazarus, a person's perception of an event is more important than the event itself. His view is called _____ because it emphasizes the importance of the combination of psychological factors (such as cognitive mediation), appraisal, vulnerability, and coping. Lazarus recognizes three kinds of appraisal—primary, secondary, and reappraisal. A person's initial judgment of an event is _____ appraisal, whereas a person's perceived ability to cope with harm, threat, or challenge is _____ appraisal. Ongoing reevaluation of the situation is _____. People who lack the resources to cope are _____. Their efforts to manage internal and external demands are called _____.

III. Sources of Stress

Although people's perception of events and their perceived ability to cope may be more important than the events themselves, several common sources of stress exist in our society.

A. Environment

Population density is a _____ condition, whereas _____ is a psychological condition stemming from many people being confined to limited space. The negative impact of these two conditions can interact with low _____ control to produce negative consequences. Low levels of personal control can also affect the stress that results from air _____, and people may react by becoming psychologically and physiologically adapted to their polluted environment. A third source of stress is _____, or noxious, unwanted auditory stimulation that intrudes into a person's environment. Although noise may be stressful, the greatest health risk of loud noise is loss of hearing. The combination of crowding, noise, pollution, commuting hassles, and fear of crime that affect city life can be referred to as _____ _____.

B. Occupation

People who have some control over their work experience have

_____ job-related stress than do either middle-level managers or people

in the services fields.

C. Personal Relationships

Personal relationships can increase or decrease stress, depending on the

_____ of the relationship. Supportive personal relationships

at work and at home are both important in buffering the potentially harmful

effects of stress.

D. Sleep Problems

The inability to fall asleep or stay asleep is called _____. In

addition, many people voluntarily deprive themselves of sleep, which may

produce psychological effects such as faulty decision-making and tension. Lack of

sleep may also have an effect on health because it decreases _____

system function.

IV. Measurement of Stress

The usefulness of stress measures rests on their ability to consistently

predict some established criterion—for example, illness.

A. Methods of Measurement

Stress has been measured by several methods. Blood pressure, heart rate, galvanic skin response, respiration rate, and biochemical measures such as cortisol and catecholamine release are some of the _____ measures used to assess stress. A disadvantage of these procedures is that the equipment and setting may themselves produce stress.

Most life events scales are patterned after the Holmes and Rahe

_____ _____ _____

_____ which is based on the premise that any major change in life is stressful. Lazarus has pioneered an alternative, a scale that measures

_____ _____ rather than major life events. The Daily Hassles Scale assumes that only unpleasant events (hassles) can be stressful and emphasizes the perceived severity of the event. Lazarus and his colleagues also published the Uplifts Scale, which assumes that uplifts or pleasant experiences will decrease stress and even promote health. The *Revised Hassles and Uplift Scale* allows people to see an event as either a hassle or an uplift

B. Reliability and Validity of Stress Measures

The reliability of self-report stress inventories can be assessed by having a person fill out the inventory more than _____. The validity of stress inventories can be established by showing a relationship between scores on the inventory and _____.

Answers

I.   neurons; neurotransmitters; synaptic; afferent; efferent; interneurons;
         central nervous; peripheral
I.A.   somatic; autonomic; sympathetic; parasympathetic; norepinephrine
I.B.   neuroendocrine; hormones; pituitary; adrenocorticotropic; adrenal; cortex;
         medulla; cortisol; epinephrine; norepinephrine
I.C.   sympathetic; neuroendocrine; glucocorticoids; epinephrine; norepinephrine
II.A.   nonspecific; General Adaptation Syndrome; alarm; exhaustion;
         psychological
II.B.   transactional; primary; secondary; reappraisal; vulnerable; coping
III.A.   physical; crowding; personal (perceived); pollution; noise; urban press
III.B.   less
III.C.   quality
III.D   insomnia; immune
IV.A.   physiological; Social Readjustment Rating Scale; daily (everyday) hassles
IV.B.   once; illness (health)

Multiple Choice Questions

_____   1. When Kyle filled out the Holmes and Rahe Social Readjustment
             Rating Scale, his score was 400. Such a score indicates that Kyle
             a. has a decreased risk for a stress-related disorder.
             b. will develop a disease during the next year.
             c. will develop a psychological disorder during the next year.
             d. has more stress than most people.

_____   2   A neuron is a(n)
             a. neurotransmitter.
             b. individual nerve cell.
             c. synapse.
             d. none of the above

_____   3. The synaptic cleft is
             a. a neuron.
             b. an individual nerve cell.
             c. the space between neurons.
             d. a group of ganglions.
             e. none of the above

_____ 4. The brain and the spinal cord are considered to be
    a. the peripheral nervous system.
    b. the central nervous system.
    c. the cardiovascular system.
    d. the somatic nervous system.

_____ 5. Sensory neurons
    a. stimulate organs and glands.
    b. are also called efferent.
    c. relay information from the sense organs to the spinal cord.
    d. all of the above

_____ 6. The two sub-divisions of the autonomic nervous system are
    a. sympathetic and parasympathetic nervous systems.
    b. the brain and the spinal cord.
    c. central and peripheral.
    d. afferents and efferents.

_____ 7. The adrenal glands are part of the _____ system.
    a. nervous
    b. cardiovascular
    c. digestive
    d. endocrine

_____ 8. Selye viewed stress as
    a. a cognitive function.
    b. a nonspecific response.
    c. a specific response.
    d. none of the above

_____ 9. Which of these is a stage of the General Adaptation Syndrome?
    a. the alarm stage
    b. the illness stage
    c. death
    d. self-efficacy

_____ 10. Which of the following has been a criticism of Selye's theory of stress?
    a. The theory places too much emphasis on emotional and psychological factors.
    b. The theory ignores physiological factors that underlie the stress response.
    c. The theory places too much emphasis on appraisal and too little on coping.
    d. The theory places too much emphasis on physiological factors and too little on psychological factors.

_____ 11. The theorist who emphasized psychological and cognitive factors in stress was
   a. Selye.
   b. Cannon.
   c. Lazarus.
   d. none of the above

_____ 12. Which of these does NOT determine a person's ability to cope with an event, according to Lazarus and Folkman?
   a. problem-solving ability
   b. the magnitude of the event itself
   c. material resources, such as money
   d. belief that one can cope with the event

_____ 13. A vulnerable person, according to Lazarus,
   a. lacks the ability to rationalize stressful situations.
   b. lacks the resources to cope with an important event.
   c. is already ill but has not yet been diagnosed.
   d. has too much ability to cope with stressful events.

_____ 14. The results of studies on crowding among rats suggest that
   a. crowding leads to early death for most rats living in such conditions.
   b. crowding leads to changes in social structure among rats.
   c. crowding causes increased fertility in rats.
   d. crowding produces no negative effects in rats.

_____ 15. In comparing crowding and density, Stokols proposed that
   a. crowding is physical and density is psychological.
   b. crowding is psychological and density is physical.
   c. both crowding and density are psychological.
   d. both crowding and density are physical.

_____ 16. During a recent basketball game, 27,000 people were in attendance. That many people in a relatively small environment would constitute
   a. overcrowding.
   b. crowding.
   c. a riot.
   d. density.

_____ 17. Which of these could be a source of stress?
   a. lack of sleep
   b. noise
   c. crowding
   d. all of the above

_____ 18. In a study of people living next to a busy street, the investigators found
   a. a positive relationship between objective noise levels and both sleep and health.
   b. a negative relationship between objective noise levels and both sleep and health.
   c. that people's subjective view of noise was related to the number of health complaints they had.
   d. both a and c

_____ 19. Urban press refers to
   a. city dwellers' flight to the suburbs.
   b. the many sources of environmental stressors that affect city living.
   c. campaigns by city newspapers that emphasize the healthy environment of the city.
   d. health-related news reports carried by the mass media.

_____ 20. With regard to the murder rate in the United States, which statement is most accurate?
   a. The murder rate has doubled every year since 1980.
   b. The murder rate has increased by about 15% per year since 1930.
   c. The murder rate has increased by about 50% per year since 1950.
   d. The murder rate was lower during the late 1990s than it was during the 1930s.

_____ 21. With regard to crime, which of these statements is most accurate?
   a. All categories of crime are on the increase in the United States.
   b. Fear of crime is related to media attention more than crime incidence.
   c. Firearm homicide rates are decreasing.
   d. Homicide and robbery rates are sharply increasing.

_____ 22. Stress-related illnesses are LEAST common among
   a. people who have jobs with high demand and low levels of control.
   b. people who have jobs with high demand and high levels of control.
   c. waiters and waitresses.
   d. construction workers.

_____ 23. People who suffer from insomnia
   a. have trouble getting to sleep.
   b. have difficulty staying asleep long enough to feel sufficiently rested.
   c. both a and b
   d. neither a nor b

_____ 24. Bryan is a high school senior who leads a busy life. He is involved in track and student government, has a part-time job, spends time with his girlfriend, and goes out with his buddies after work. He has been having trouble concentrating in class and in track practice. The most likely explanation for Bryan's condition is
    a. stress from the pollution and noise of the city in which he lives.
    b. a sudden onset of paranoia.
    c. sleep deprivation.
    d. stress from his impending graduation and the life changes that will accompany his future life.

_____ 25. Health psychologists are most likely to use these instruments to measure stress.
    a. performance tests
    b. physiological measures
    c. self-report scales
    d. reports of significant others

_____ 26. This scale assumes that changes in life adjustment is the key factor in measuring stress.
    a. the Social Readjustment Rating Scale
    b. the Daily Hassles Scale
    c. the Uplift Scale
    d. the Perceived Stress Scale

_____ 27. This scale allows people to rate an everyday event either positively or negatively.
    a. the Social Readjustment Rating Scale
    b. the revised Daily Hassles and Uplifts Scale
    c. the Perceived Stress Scale
    d. all of the above

_____ 28. One way of determining the reliability of a stress inventory is to have people fill out the inventory twice. Another method is to compare participants' scores with
    a. scores of spouses who filled out the inventory from the participant's point of view.
    b. the number of illnesses per person per year.
    c. scores on the Social Readjustment Rating Scale.
    d. the number of people who take the stress inventory.

_____ 29. The validity of self-report inventories is complicated by this question:
     a.   What should the scale measure?
     b.   How high should the reliability be?
     c.   What physiology underlies the stress response?
     d.   What physiological factors underlie stress?

_____ 30. The MOST important attribute of a stress inventory is its
     a.   reliability.
     b.   ability to test hypothetical assumptions underlying a given theory of stress.
     c.   standardization.
     d.   ability to predict illness.

Multiple Choice Answers

1.	d		16.	d
2.	b		17.	d
3.	c		18.	c
4.	b		19.	b
5.	c		20.	d
6.	a		21.	b
7.	d		22.	b
8.	b		23.	c
9.	a		24.	c
10.	d		25.	c
11.	c		26.	a
12.	b		27.	b
13.	b		28.	a
14.	b		29.	a
15.	b		30.	d

Physiology of the Stress Response

Fill in the blanks to complete the correct responses for the neuroendocrine and autonomic nervous system activation during stress.

In the brain

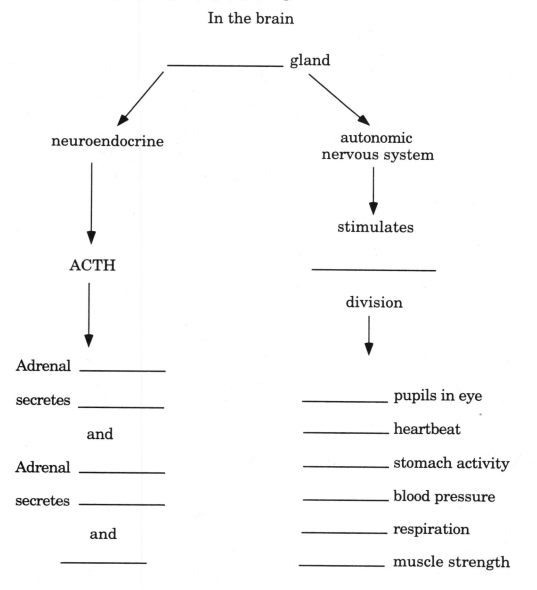

_____ gland

neuroendocrine   autonomic nervous system

ACTH   stimulates

                              _____

                              division

Adrenal _____

secretes _____   _____ pupils in eye

and   _____ heartbeat

Adrenal _____   _____ stomach activity

secretes _____   _____ blood pressure

and   _____ respiration

_____   _____ muscle strength

Essay Questions

1. Franklin is a college sophomore majoring in premed. He has made 67% on his first exam in anatomy. Analyze Franklin's response to this event in terms of Lazarus's theory of stress, including appraisal and vulnerability.

2. How does the factor of personal control influence the stress related to crowding, noise, pollution, and urban life?

Good points to include in your essay answers:

1. A. Franklin would go through the process of appraisal, including primary
    and secondary appraisal and reappraisal.
    1. His primary appraisal would be his initial perception of the low grade
    in terms of stressful, irrelevant, or benign-positive. A primary appraisal
    of *stressful* is likely because Franklin would probably perceive a low grade
    as harmful, threatening, or challenging to his current grade point average
    and thus to his medical career.
    2. Franklin's secondary appraisal would include his evaluation of his
    ability to cope with the low grade. He might consider how many other
    tests and how well he thinks he can do on other work for the course.
    3. Reappraisal includes reevaluations of the situation, which may
    decrease or increase stress. Franklin may experience reduced stress if he
    finds that others in the class also did poorly, leading the instructor to
    "curve" the grades. His stress might be increased by good performance by
    his classmates or by the importance of this exam for his final grade.
    B. Franklin's vulnerability will be determined by his perception of his ability
    to cope with the grade.
    1. He may feel vulnerable and stressed because he studied and believes
    that he did as well as he can.
    2. He may feel less vulnerable because he believes that he can improve
    his grade.

2. A. Lack of control may interact with crowding to produce the negative
    health effects of crowding.
    1. The ability to control noise leads to the perception of the noise as less
    stressful.
    2. Pollution tends to be beyond personal control, which may lead to a
    feeling of helplessness and acceptance.
    3. The urban environment includes commuting hassles and fear of crime
    in addition to crowding, pollution, and noise, and these urban stressors
    are beyond personal control.
    B. A feeling of personal control may mediate the stress of crowding,
    pollution, noise, and urban life, either adding to the stress by a feeling of lack
    of control or buffering stress with a perception of control.

Let's Get Personal—
Assess Your Stress

You can assess your stress by taking the Social Readjustment Rating Scale (SRRS), which appears as the Check Your Health Risks box at the beginning of this chapter. Fill it out and add your stress points to determine your score.

Was your score high enough to indicate that you are in danger of becoming ill? What is the score that represents an elevated risk?

Do you think that the SRRS captured the stresses of your life?

What questions were inappropriate for you?

What areas of stress did the SRRS miss?

Do you think that the Daily Hassles Scale would be more appropriate to reflect the stress in your life?

Understanding Stress and Disease

Fill in the Rest of the Story

I. Physiology of the Immune System

The immune system consists of tissues, organs, and processes that protect the body from invasion by foreign material such as bacteria, _____ and fungi. It also removes worn-out or damaged cells from the body.

A. Organs of the Immune System

The immune system includes lymph, a circulating fluid that contains a type of white blood cell called _____. Various types of lymphocytes include T-cells, B-cells, and _____ _____ (NK) cells.

B. Function of the Immune System

The immune system defends the body against foreign invaders through both specific and nonspecific responses. Specific immunity is called _____ - _____ immunity, and those substances manufactured in response to a specific invader are called _____. After the invaders have been destroyed, the immune system keeps the critical information that allows future manufacture of antibodies, creating _____ to the invader that can persist for years.

C. Immune System Disorders

Examples of the immune system's failure to protect a person include acquired immune deficiency syndrome (AIDS), allergies, and

_____ disorders that originate from the immune system's failure to distinguish body cells from invaders and results in an attack on one's own body cells.

II. Psychoneuroimmunology

The interdisciplinary field that focuses on the interactions among behavior, the nervous system, the endocrine system, and the immune system is called

_____. Research in psychoneuroimmunology has attempted to reveal the interactions among behavior, the _____ system, the _____ system, and the immune system by demonstrating that behavior can affect the immune system and that illness can result from these effects.

A. History of Psychoneuroimmunology

In 1974, Robert Ader and Nicholas Cohen demonstrated that the immune system could be _____ and thus began the field of psychoneuroimmunology.

B. Research in Psychoneuroimmunology

Research has demonstrated that behavior can _____ immune system function, and a depressed immune system function relates to subsequent

_____. Research in the field of psychoneuroimmunology has

demonstrated the sequence of _____ immune system depression,

and disease.

C. Physical Mechanisms of Influence

The link between behavior and depressed immune function must occur

through some physical mechanism. Researchers have looked at both the action of

the peripheral nervous system during stress and neuroendocrine responses in the

_____.

D. Therapeutic Effects

Although research has clearly shown that behavior can suppress immune

system function, data exist indicating that behavioral interventions can

_____ immune system function.

III. Does Stress Cause Disease?

Stress is one of many factors that may cause illness, but in general, it adds

only a _____ risk and that risk is usually temporary.

A. Stress and Disease

Because stress responses can act in many ways throughout the body, it has

potential to cause _____ damage and contribute to such

disorders as headaches, infectious illness, cardiovascular disease, and other

physiological illnesses. Stress may contribute to both tension and

_____ headaches, the two most common types of headache.

Research that involved exposing people to _____ viruses has shown that stress is an important factor in vulnerability to infectious illness. The relationship between stress and cardiovascular disease is complex and not well-established. Stress has a stronger influence on temporary increases in blood pressure than on chronic hypertension. The tendency for some people to react more strongly than other people to stress is called _____. Hostility, coping style, gender, and ethnic background all relate to reactivity; that is, increased blood pressure, _____ rate, and other biological responses.

B. Stress and Negative Mood

Stress also relates to _____ affectivity; that is, the tendency to experience distress and dissatisfaction in a variety of situations. Because of this link, it may contribute to depress and anxiety, although the evidence for such a causal link is not great. Currently, researchers believe that stress is neither a necessary nor a _____ ingredient in the development of depression. Anxiety disorders include panic attack, agoraphobia, generalized anxiety, obsessive-compulsive disorders, and _____

_____ disorder (PTSD). PTSD is, by definition, related to stress, but stress is less clearly related to the other anxiety disorders.

IV. Personality Factors Affecting Stress and Illness

Because stress seems to affect some people more than it does others, researchers have looked for personality variables and have formulated several

models that might account for differential effects of stress. One such model

suggests that some individuals are vulnerable to stress-related illnesses because

either genetic weakness or biochemical imbalance inherently predispose them to

those illnesses. This model, called the _____ -

_____ model, assumes a person must have a relatively permanent

predisposition to the illness and must experience some sort of stress that

precipitates the illness. An alternate formulation, called the

_____ personality model, hypothesizes that hardy individuals

have a strong sense of _____ to self, demonstrate an internal

locus of control, and are likely to see necessary adjustments as a

_____.

Answers

I.   viruses
I.A.   lymphocytes; natural killer
I.B.   cell-mediated; antibodies; immunity
I.C.   autoimmune
II.   psychoneuroimmunology; endocrine; nervous
II.A.   conditioned
II.B.   depress; disease (illness); behavior
II.C.   brain
II.D.   boost
III.   moderate (slight)
III.A.   organic (physiological); migraine; respiratory (cold or rhino); reactivity; heart
III.B.   negative; sufficient; posttraumatic stress
IV.   diatheses-stress; hardy; commitment; challenge

Multiple Choice Questions

_____ 1. The system whose main function is to defend the body against foreign invaders is the
  a. endocrine system.
  b. autonomic nervous system.
  c. somatic nervous system.
  d. immune system.

_____ 2. Which of these is an organ of the immune system?
  a. liver
  b. heart
  c. tonsils
  d. bronchi

_____ 3. If the body were a kingdom, the immune system would be the
  a. king.
  b. court jester.
  c. army.
  d. heir to the throne.

_____ 4. The function of antibodies is to
  a. create leukocytes.
  b. produce immunity.
  c. promote memory T-cells.
  d. divide T-cells from B-cells.

_____ 5. HIV is caused by
  a. homosexuality.
  b. injection drug use.
  c. a virus.
  d. a bacterium.
  e. all of the above

_____ 6. Psychoneuroimmunology is a relatively new discipline dealing primarily with
  a. the causes of HIV.
  b. the cure for AIDS.
  c. the interactions among behavior, the endocrine system, the immune system, and the nervous system.
  d. the interactions among behavior, the cardiovascular system, the immune system, the nervous system, and stress.

_____ 7. Research suggests that immunity can be enhanced by
  a. people writing about their traumatic experiences.
  b. relaxation training.
  c. aerobic training.
  d. all of the above
  e. none of the above

_____ 8. The notion that some people are more inherently vulnerable to the effects of stress than are other people is called
  a. the hardiness hypothesis.
  b. the identity disruption model.
  c. psychoneuroimmunology.
  d. the diathesis-stress model.

_____ 9. The theory that holds that psychologically healthy people are buffered against the harmful effects of stress is
  a. the identity disruption model.
  b. the diathesis-stress model.
  c. the personal hardiness model.
  d. the Type A model.

_____ 10. Which of these is NOT a component of Kobasa's hardiness concept?
  a. cooperation
  b. commitment
  c. challenge
  d. control

_____ 11. If stress causes illness, then this system most likely plays a central role in that process.
  a. nervous
  b. digestive
  c. cardiovascular
  d. immune

_____ 12. Evidence is most clear for a relationship between stress and
  a. ulcers.
  b. Alzheimer's disease.
  c. decreased immune function.
  d. cancer.

_____ 13. The term reactivity means that some people
  a. respond more strongly to stress than do other people.
  b. respond with more intense anger than do other people.
  c. respond more quickly to fearful stimuli than do other people.
  d. all of the above

_____ 14. This personality variable is most reliability related to reactivity.
    a. hostility
    b. Type A behavior pattern
    c. Type B behavior pattern
    d. extraversion
    e. introversion

_____ 15. A synergistic effect exists whenever the combination of two factors
    a. produces a greater effect than the sum of those two factors.
    b. creates a diminished effect compared to the sum of the two factors.
    c. produces an effect that is less than either of the two factors.
    d. none of the above

_____ 16. The relationship among smoking, stress, and illness is complicated by the possibility that
    a. stress may increase the amount of smoking a person does.
    b. smokers may use smoking a coping mechanism rather than finding healthy ways of coping.
    c. stress and smoking may have a synergistic effect on illness.
    d. any of the above

_____ 17. With regard to gender and stress, which of these statements is FALSE?
    a. Stressed men are more likely to drink heavily than stressed women.
    b. Stressed women are more likely to use illicit drugs than stressed men.
    c. Stressed women are more likely to change their eating patterns than stressed men.
    d. All the statements are true.

_____ 18. Contrary to popular belief, stress is a minor factor in the development of
    a. rheumatoid arthritis.
    b. headache.
    c. asthma.
    d. ulcers.

_____ 19. Stress during pregnancy is most likely to result in
    a. spontaneous abortions.
    b. underweight babies.
    c. multiple births.
    d. all of the above

_____ 20. Stress is most likely to relate to depression when a person
   a. is vulnerable but has strong coping skills.
   b. is not vulnerable but has poor coping skills.
   c. is vulnerable and has poor coping skills.
   d. is highly stressed but has no perception of stress.

_____ 21. Stressful life events correlate with depression
   a. positively and strongly.
   b. positively but weakly.
   c. negatively and strongly.
   d. negatively but weakly.

_____ 22. Charlotte suffers from recurrent memories that intrude into her
   thoughts. She also has unpleasant dreams that replay a distressing
   experienced of being mugged and robbed three years ago. The
   extreme psychological and physiological distress she experiences best
   fits the definition of
   a. posttraumatic stress disorder.
   b. clinical depression.
   c. schizophrenia.
   d. transcendent psychosis.

_____ 23. The person who is most likely to experience a stress-related disorder
   is one who
   a. has a diathesis that protects against stress.
   b. feels low in personal control.
   c. has an executive position that requires many decisions.
   d. has relatives who have experienced stress-related disorders
       during adolescence.

_____ 24. Garland has been healthy for the past year. What does his good
   health reveal about his level of stress?
   a. He has a low level of stress.
   b. He has a high level of stress but good coping abilities.
   c. He has a supportive wife who provides a relationship in which he
       can be emotionally expressive.
   d. Nothing—the relationship between stress and illness is far from
       perfect.

Multiple Choice Answers

1.	d	13.	a
2.	c	14.	a
3.	c	15.	a
4.	b	16.	d
5.	c	17.	b
6.	c	18.	d
7.	d	19.	b
8.	d	20.	c
9.	c	21.	b
10.	a	22.	a
11.	d	23	b
12	c	24.	d

Match the researchers with their research:

1. Robert Ader and Nicholas Cohen

   a. formulated the hardy personality model.

2. Barry Marshall and J. Robin Warren

   b. demonstrated that stress plays a role in vulnerability to infectious illness.

3. Suzanne Kobasa

   c. demonstrated that immune response is lowered by psychological stress.

4. Janice Kiecolt-Glaser and Ronald Glaser

   d. demonstrated that a bacterium and not stress is the cause of most ulcers.

5. Sheldon Cohen

   e. demonstrated that the immune system can be classically conditioned.

1. e   2. d   3. a   4. c   5. b

Immune Response

Fill in the missing information to complete the sequence of events for the primary immune response. How does the time frame compare to that of the secondary immune response?

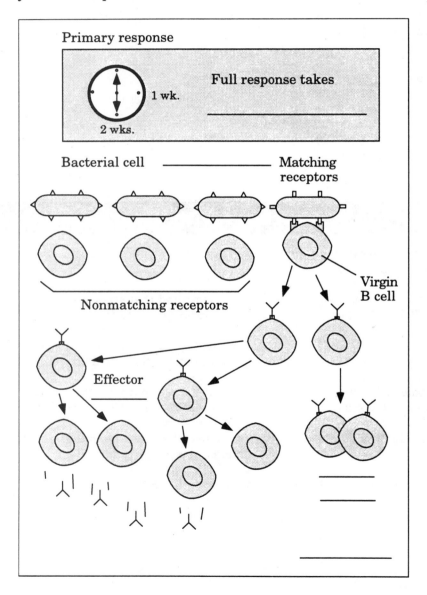

Primary response

Full response takes

1 wk.

2 wks.

Bacterial cell _____ Matching receptors

Nonmatching receptors

Virgin B cell

Effector

Essay Questions

1. What happens when the immune system begins to lose its effectiveness? How can this loss occur?

2. Which physical illnesses have a strong stress component? For which is the evidence less clear?

CHAPTER 6 / STRESS AND DISEASE 97

Good points to include in your essay answers:

1. A. When the immune system loses its effectiveness, the body becomes vulnerable to wide variety of viral, bacterial, fungal, and parasitic invaders.
    1. Impairment off nonspecific immune blocks tissue repair, because inflammation and phagocytosis will not occur, leaving the body vulnerable to infection by these invaders.
    2. Impairment of specific immune function impairs the formation of antibodies, which attack specific invaders; this deficit would prevent the formation of immunity.
    3. With impaired immune system function, attempts at immunization could be dangerous, because immunization typically occurs through the introduction of weakened forms of the disease; without the ability to form antibodies, these weakened pathogens could cause disease.
   B. Immune deficiency occurs both as an inherent condition and as the result of infection with the human immunodeficiency virus.
    1. Children born without functional immune systems must remain isolated from pathogens or they will die from exposure to the many diseases that most people can withstand.
    2. People infected with HIV lose their immune function and die from one of the many infections that their bodies can no longer fight.

2. A. Stress is a factor in both vascular and tension headaches.
   B. Stress is related to vulnerability to infectious illness.
   C. The relationship between stress and cardiovascular disease is not straightforward, but some people show high levels of reactivity or sodium retention when under stress, which may be a factor in the development of cardiovascular disease.
   D. Other disorders such as diabetes, premature delivery in pregnancy, asthma, and rheumatoid arthritis are related to stress, but the exact role of stress in the development of these diseases is not clear.
   E. Evidence exists that stress is related to physical disorders, but the evidence is less clear than most people assume.

Let's Get Personal—

Headache Analysis

Do you have headaches that relate to the stress in your life? Headaches are the disorder with the strongest relationship to stress, and most people experience headaches at some times. Tension, migraine, and cluster headaches all have some stress component.

To analyze the relationship between your stress and headaches, keep a headache diary for at least a week. Note your headaches, time of day, and activities that preceded each one. To what extent was some stressful event or combination of events responsible for triggering the headaches? How did you cope with your headaches, and did these coping techniques address the stress component?

For each day and for each headache, furnish the following information:

Time of Headache—

What I was doing when I noticed I had a headache—

Was stress a factor in this triggering this headache?

If so, what was the stressful event?

What I did when I noticed I had a headache—

This action worked to alleviate my headache by—

CHAPTER 7
Understanding Pain

Fill in the Rest of the Story

I. Pain and the Nervous System

All sensory stimulation, including pain, starts with activation of sensory neurons and proceeds with the relay of neural impulses toward the

_____.

A. Somatosensory System

The _____ system conveys sensory information from the body through the spinal cord to the brain. Sensory or _____ neurons convey information from sense organs toward the brain. Primary afferents are those neurons that have receptors in the sense organs. They originate the electrochemical neural message, beginning with _____ potentials. The vast number of neurons and their interconnections makes neural transmission complex and difficult to envision.

Three different types of neurons are involved with transmitting pain impulses. The large _____ - _____ fibers and smaller _____ - _____ fibers are covered with a protective covering called _____, which speeds neural transmission. The smaller and more common _____ fibers require high levels of stimulation to fire.

99

B. The Spinal Cord

Primary afferents from the skin enter the _____

_____ where they synapse with secondary afferents called

_____ cells in the dorsal horns of the spinal cord. The dorsal

horns contain several layers called _____, and laminae 1 and 2

form a structure called the _____ _____ that

receives sensory input from the A and C fibers. Complex interactions of sensory

input occur in the laminae of the dorsal horns, and these interactions may affect

the perception of sensory input before it gets to the brain.

C. The Brain

The brain structure that receives sensory input from the different neural

tracts in the spinal cord is the _____. The skin is mapped in the

somatosensory cortex in the _____ lobe of the cerebral cortex, and

the proportion of cortex devoted to an area of skin is proportional to that skin's

sensitivity to stimulation. Sensory information from internal organs are not

mapped as precisely as the skin.

D. Neurotransmitters and Pain

The neurotransmitters that form the basis for neural transmission also play

a role in pain perception. The discovery of the endogenous opiates—enkephalin,

_____ , and dynorphin—led to the discovery of neural receptors

specialized for these neurotransmitters and the conclusion that opiate drugs produce analgesia because of the brain's own chemistry. The neurotransmitters serotonin and substance P and the chemicals brandykinin and prostaglandins may exacerbate pain perception.

E. The Modulation of Pain

When a structure in the midbrain is stimulated, pain relief occurs. This structure is called the _____ _____. The neurons in the periaqueductal gray synapse with neurons in a structure in the medulla called the _____ _____

_____. These neurons descend to the spinal cord and may constitute a descending control system for pain perception.

II. The Meaning of Pain

Most researchers see pain as having two dimensions, an organic component and a psychological or emotional component, and the experience of pain is usually linked to both dimensions.

A. The Stages of Pain

At least three stages of pain have been identified. The type of pain that is ordinarily adaptive, lasts a relatively short period of time, and includes pain from cuts, burns, and other physical trauma is _____ pain. When pain endures beyond the time of normal healing, is relatively constant, is often reinforced by other people, and becomes self-perpetuating, it is called

_____. Pain experienced between acute and chronic pain is called

_____. This intermediate time is critical because during this time the pain may either terminate or evolve into chronic pain.

B. Pain Syndromes

Pain can be classified according to location or syndrome. Headaches are the most frequent pain syndrome in the United States. The most common varieties are migraine, tension, and cluster headaches. _____ (or vascular) headaches bring about loss of appetite, nausea, vomiting, and increased sensitivity to light. Those headaches caused by contractions of the muscles of the neck, shoulders, scalp, and face are _____ headaches. Headaches that produce intense pain localized in one side of the head and occur frequently over a period of days are _____ headaches.

Another common pain syndrome is low back pain, which has many causes. The most common cause of low back pain is injury, but _____ and other psychological factors may be involved. People with low back pain may be exempt from unpleasant tasks, which can perpetuate their pain behaviors and prevent their recovery.

A variety of arthritic pains exist, and many involve inflammation of the joints. Perhaps the most frequent cause of arthritic pain is an autoimmune disorder called _____ _____, which is characterized by a dull ache within or around a joint. A progressive inflammation of the joints that is characterized by a dull ache in the joint area and tends to affect older people is called _____. Cancer pain is present in about two-thirds

of all cancer cases. Cancer pain may be caused by either the cancer itself or by

the _____ of the cancer. Amputees nearly always continue to feel

some sensation in the missing body part, and the feeling is frequently painful.

This experience of chronic pain in an amputated part of the body is known as

_____ _____ _____.

C. Theories of Pain

Pain is a complex phenomenon that is not completely understood, giving rise

to several theories of pain. The leading model of pain is the _____

_____ theory proposed by Ronald Melzack and Peter Wall. This theory

hypothesizes that a gating mechanism exists in the _____

_____, specifically in the structure called the

_____ _____ of the dorsal horns of the spinal

cord. This modulation can change pain perception, as can brain-level alterations

from a hypothesized _____ _____ trigger. This

theory includes explanations of both physiological and psychological modulations

of the pain experience. Melzack has proposed an extension to the gate control

theory that puts an even stronger emphasis on the brain's role in pain perception,

an extension called _____ theory.

III. The Measurement of Pain

A number of techniques have been used to measure laboratory and clinical pain, and these fall into three main categories: physiological measures, behavioral assessments, and self-reports.

A. Physiological Measures

Several physiological variables have potential to measure pain, including muscle tension and autonomic indices. Muscle tension as measured by _____ (EMG) has an inconsistent relationship with perceived pain severity, but autonomic indices such as skin temperature show some promise.

B. Behavioral Assessment

Health psychologists generally have preferred observation of _____ to assess pain, looking at the ways that people in pain communicate to others and the reinforcements that pain can bring. Significant others, such as spouses, can be trained to make observations of pain behaviors without reinforcing them.

C. Self-Reports

Self-report measures of pain include rating scales, standardized pain inventories, and standardized _____ inventories. With rating scales, patients are asked to rate the intensity of their pain on a scale—for example, from 1 to 100. Melzack developed an inventory that categorizes pain into sensory, affective, and evaluative dimensions. This inventory is called the _____ Pain Inventory. A more recent attempt to assess pain, the

West Haven Yale Multidimensional Pain Inventory, can reliably classify pain sufferers into three clusters: (1) those who cope poorly and whose pain interferes with their lives, labeled _____; (2) those who are upset because they feel that they receive little support, labeled _____ distressed; and (3) those who are more active and less distressed by their pain, called _____ copers. Standardized tests, such as the Minnesota Multiphasic Personality Inventory (MMPI), have also been used to assess pain and have some ability to differentiate among types of pain patients.

IV. Preventing Pain

Preventing pain is preferable to waiting for pain to occur and then treating it. The two main methods of preventing pain are (1) minimizing injuries and (2) preventing acute pain from becoming _____ pain.

V. Physical Treatments for Pain

Medical treatments are used for both acute and _____ types of pain, but pain patients may not receive adequate medication because medical personnel tend to _____ patients' pain.

A. Drugs

The most common treatment for acute pain are _____ drugs. These drugs are usually either of the aspirin type or the opiate type. Aspirin is one of the _____ _____ - _____ drugs (NSAIDs). Along with ibuprofen and naproxen sodium, these drugs are useful in managing minor pain, but more powerful analgesic effects can be obtained from

_____, but the fear that this drug will cause addiction and other

drug-related problems prevents many physicians from prescribing it.

B. Skin Stimulation

Electrical stimulation of the skin can produce analgesic effects, and devices

that produce transcutaneous electrical _____ stimulation (TENS)

began to be used for both acute and chronic pain during the 1970s. Patients with

both acute and chronic pain can use TENS to achieve relief. The ancient Chinese

form of analgesia that consists of inserting needles into the skin and

manipulating the needles is called _____. Although its success

is due to more than the placebo effect, acupuncture alone is rarely sufficient to

produce a high degree of analgesia. Other methods of skin stimulation include

_____, which uses pressure rather than needles, and massage,

which involves the direct manipulation of soft tissue.

C. Surgery

The most drastic form of treatment for chronic pain is _____,

but it is often unsuccessful in alleviating chronic pain and often produces

additional unwanted effects.

D. Limitations of Physical Treatments

Medical treatment is the first choice for _____ pain, but it has

been less successful with chronic pain. The most effective analgesic drugs are of the _____ type, but their potential for abuse has made health care

professionals reluctant to prescribe adequate doses. Ironically, the best

treatment may be no treatment. One study indicated that people who received

no treatment recovered faster than those who were restricted to

_____ rest or who performed back exercises.

Answers

I.   brain
I.A.   somatosensory; afferent; action; A-beta; A-delta; myelin; C
I.B.   spinal cord; transmission; laminae; substantia gelatinosa
I.C.   thalamus; parietal
I.D.   endorphin
I.E.   periaqueductal gray; nucleus raphé magnus
II.A.   acute; chronic; prechronic
II.B.   Migraine; tension; cluster; stress; rheumatoid arthritis; osteoarthritis; treatment; phantom limb pain
II.C.   gate control; spinal cord; substantia gelatinosa; central control; neuromatrix
III.A. electromyograph
III.B. behavior
III.C. personality; McGill; dysfunctional; interpersonally; adaptive
IV.   chronic
V.   chronic; underestimate (minimize)
V.A.   analgesic; nonsteroidal anti-inflammatory; opiates
V.B.   nerve; acupuncture; acupressure
V.C.   surgery
V.D.   acute; opiate; bed

Multiple Choice Questions

_____ ·   1. Throughout the world, about _____ % of the people suffer from some
            type of persistent, chronic pain.
            a. 7%
            b. 20%
            c. 35%
            d. 50%

_____   2. The _____ system permits people to interpret certain sensory
            information as pain.
            a. muscular
            b. skeletal
            c. endocrine
            d. somatosensory

_____   3. Sensory impulses are conveyed directly to the spinal cord by
            a. primary afferents.
            b. secondary afferents.
            c. the peripheral nervous system.
            d. motor neurons.

_____   4. The dorsal horns are located on the
            a. midbrain.
            b. myelin.
            c. spinal cord.
            d. brain stem.

_____   5. The substantia gelatinosa
            a. connects afferent neurons to efferent neurons.
            b. receives information from the efferent system.
            c. is capable of modulating sensory input.
            d. none of the above

_____   6. Alice has just smashed her finger with a hammer. She experiences
            _____ pain.
            a. chronic
            b. chronic intractable
            c. prechronic
            d. acute

_____ 7. Which of these is a distinction between chronic and acute pain?
   a. Chronic pain is usually adaptive; acute pain is not.
   b. Acute pain has a cause; chronic pain does not.
   c. Chronic pain is often prolonged by environmental reinforcers; acute pain needs no such reinforcement.
   d. Chronic pain warns us to avoid further injury; acute pain has no such warning ability.

_____ 8. In the United States, more people suffer from this type of pain than from any other.
   a. low back pain
   b. headache
   c. acute
   d. chronic recurrent

_____ 9. Odessa experiences recurrent pain that is accompanied by sensitivity to light, loss of appetite, and nausea. The most likely diagnosis is
   a. tension headaches.
   b. migraine headaches.
   c. low back pain.
   d. phantom limb pain.

_____ 10. Preston is a 45-year-old librarian who has never experienced a migraine headache. His chances of a first migraine are
   a. very low.
   b. about one in five.
   c. about 50/50.
   d. very high.

_____ 11. A psychologist working with a man experiencing low back pain should recognize that
   a. the pain may be phantom limb pain.
   b. the patient's friends and family members may be reinforcing his pain behaviors.
   c. the cause of the pain is most likely psychosomatic.
   d. the patients must maintain proper posture and avoid those situations that will aggravate tissue damage.

_____ 12. Carter suffers from low back pain. Research from Finland indicates that Carter should
   a. avoid lifting any weight more than five pounds.
   b. rest in bed until the pain gets better.
   c. work out with heavy weights, that is, weight over 50 pounds.
   d. go about his regular activities.

_____ 13. Rheumatoid arthritis, unlike osteoarthritis,
   a. is an autoimmune disorder.
   b. occurs only in elderly people.
   c. often develops into chronic pain.
   d. all of the above

_____ 14. Phantom limb pain
   a. is the same as stump pain.
   b. does not occur in women who have had a breast removed.
   c. increases in frequency as time goes by.
   d. none of the above

_____ 15. This theory of pain assumes that a person's experience of pain is virtually equal to the degree of tissue damage:
   a. specificity theory.
   b. sensory decision theory.
   c. the gate control theory.
   d. all of the above

_____ 16. The gate control theory of pain was proposed by
   a. Bonica.
   b. Lazarus.
   c. Melzack and Wall.
   d. Turk and Meichenbaum.

_____ 17. The gate control theory of pain assumes that
   a. the spinal cord modulates the input of sensory information.
   b. the cerebellum is mostly responsible for the sensation of pain.
   c. individual perception is mostly responsible for the feeling of pain.
   d. classical conditioning experiences are largely responsible for the sensation of pain.

_____ 18. Marcie's husband is constantly complaining about pain in his lower back. He also walks with a limp and moans audibly when he is near Marcie. To help her husband, Marcie should
   a. ignore her husband's complaints, limps, and moans.
   b. seek medical treatment for her husband.
   c. give her husband daily back massages.
   d. do all the heavy lifting in her house.

_____ 19. Observing and measuring pain-related behaviors is most compatible with
   a.   classical conditioning.
   b.   operant conditioning.
   c.   transactional analysis.
   d.   analytical psychology.

_____ 20. In general, judgments of observers trained to identify pain behaviors
   a.   are unreliable.
   b.   are moderately reliable.
   c.   are highly reliable.
   d.   are somewhat reliable but have no validity.

_____ 21. Which of these pain assessing instruments yields these three clusters of pain patients: adaptive copers, interpersonally distressed, and dysfunctional?
   a.   the Visual Analog Scale
   b.   the West Haven-Yale Multidimensional Pain Inventory
   c.   the McGill Pain Questionnaire
   d.   The Minnesota Multiphasic Personality Inventory

_____ 22. This type of medication includes aspirin and ibuprofen:
   a.   nonsteroidal anti-inflammatory drugs.
   b.   acetaminophens.
   c.   opiate drugs.
   d.   none of the above

_____ 23. Opiate drugs
   a.   are not effective analgesics.
   b.   can produce dependence.
   c.   do not produce tolerance.
   d.   all of the above

_____ 24. Studies of diverse cultures show that
   a. African American patients receive less analgesic medication than do European American patients.
   b. pain experiences during childbirth are quite uniform throughout the world.
   c. Italian Americans in pain express less distress than do other European Americans.
   d. Chinese, compared with Europeans, consider cancer pain to be a more serious problem.

_____ 25. As a treatment for pain, acupuncture
   a. is more effective than a placebo.
   b. is no more effective than a placebo.
   c. cannot produce analgesia in animals.
   d. is effective among Chinese but not Europeans.

Multiple Choice Answers

1.	b		14.	d
2.	d		15.	a
3.	a		16	c
4.	c		17.	a
5.	c		18.	a
6.	d		19	b
7.	c		20	c
8.	b		21.	b
9.	b		22.	a
10.	a		23.	b
11.	b		24.	a
12.	d		25.	a
13.	a			

Opening and Closing the Gate

Fill in the missing information to represent the gate control mechanism in both the open and closed positions.

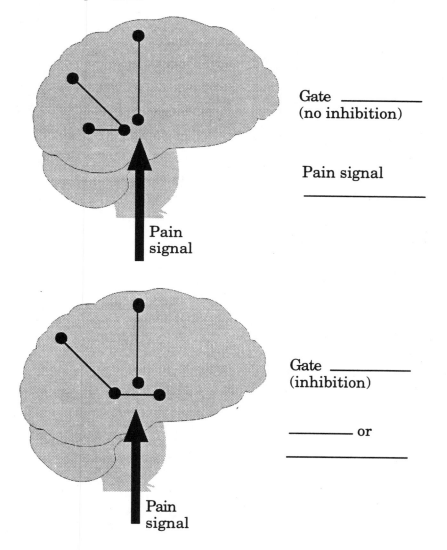

Gate _____
(no inhibition)

Pain signal

_____

Gate _____
(inhibition)

_____ or

_____

Pain
signal

Pain
signal

Essay Questions

1. Bryan cut his ankle. What could decrease his experience of the pain resulting from the cut?

2. What are the advantages and disadvantages of the various physical treatments for pain?

Good points to include in your essay answers:

1. A. If Bryan has a congenital insensitivity to pain, then the cut did not hurt, but this situation is very unlikely.
   B. Bryan's pain would probably be decreased if
   1. he was involved with some other distracting activity when the cut occurred.
   2. he was not looking at his ankle when the injury occurred.
   3. he did not look at his ankle after the cut so that he did not see the extent of his injury.
   4. he pressed tightly on the cut, stimulating other neurons in addition to the ones carrying pain messages and partially blocking the pain.
   5. he experienced some other injury in another part of his body, producing another type and location of pain.
   6. he believed that men should not be bothered by minor injuries or that he was the type of man who should not feel pain by such an injury.

2. A. Each of the physical treatments for pain has both advantages and disadvantages.
   B. Analgesic drug treatments are common.
   1. Nonsteroidal anti-inflammatory drugs (NSAIDs) and other over-the-counter analgesics can be effective for acute pain and sometimes for chronic pain.
   2. Opiate drugs are very successful in relieving severe pain, but they produce tolerance and dependence, creating the potential for abuse and making these drugs unsuitable for the management of chronic pain.
   C. Surgery is less common than analgesic drugs and less successful.
   1. Severing nerves can prevent pain messages from reaching the brain, but all surgery carries hazards.
   2. Any effect, including unpleasant ones, will be permanent.
   3. Surgery usually does not produce relief from chronic pain.
   D. TENS works by applying electrical stimulation to the skin, which produces analgesic effects., but the relief is temporary.
   E. Acupuncture and acupressure work by stimulating pressure points, either with needles inserted into the skin or pressure applied to the skin.
   1. Produce analgesic effects that are not due to the placebo effect but may not be very strong for some people.
   2. Is growing in popularity, along with other alternative therapies.
   F. Massage also involves manipulation of the skin and can be therapeutic, but its effects do not persist longer than the therapy

Let's Get Personal—

Charting Your Pain

Except people with chronic pain insensitivity, everyone experiences pain. For most people, acute pain is a common but not a serious event. For others, chronic pain is part of their lives every day. To help understand your pain, keep a pain diary for at least a week and preferably for longer.

Record the following information, and after keeping a record of your pain experience for at least a week, decide what role pain plays in your life

Day—

Time of day—

Source of the pain—

Severity of the pain—

Barely   Worst Pain
Painful   Imaginable

1   2   3   4   5   6   7   8   9   10

I coped with the pain by

Other people did / did not know that I was in pain because I

Those people who knew I was in pain reacted by

This pain caused me to make the following changes in my daily routine—

CHAPTER 8
Coping with Stress and Pain

Fill in the Rest of the Story

I. Personal Resources That Influence Coping

Humans have a natural tendency toward health and away from distress, disease, and pain. When these problems become part of our lives, we attempt to restore health through a variety of _____ techniques. At least two important personal resources influence people's ability to cope.

A. Social Support

The personal resource that includes the emotional quality of one's social contacts is called _____ _____. In general, people with high levels of social support, as compared with those with low levels, are only about _____ as likely to die within a designated period of time. Marriage provides social support, but _____ seem to profit more than _____ from marriage, and they seem to be at increased risk from the death of a spouse. Women profit more from other sources of social support, perhaps due to their tendency to have larger social _____. Social support may contribute to good health because (1) people with good social support receive more encouragement and advice to seek _____ care, and (2) social support itself may provide a

_____ against disease. Neither of these two suggestions has been strongly supported by research.

B. Personal Control

A second personal resource is one's feelings of personal control. When people are allowed to assume even small amounts of personal control and _____, they seem to live longer and have healthier lives.

II. Techniques of Coping with Stress and Pain

Health professionals have used a number of nonmedical interventions to help people cope with pain and stress, including relaxation training, hypnotic treatment, biofeedback, behavior modification, and cognitive therapy.

A. Relaxation Training

Health psychologists frequently use one or more relaxation techniques to manage stress and pain. These techniques include: (1) progressive _____ relaxation, (2) mediative relaxation, (3) mindfulness meditation, and (4) guided _____. With _____ muscle relaxation, patients learn to relax the entire body, one muscle group at a time, and to breathe deeply and exhale slowly. The type of relaxation in which muscle relaxation is combined with a quiet environment, a repetitive sound, and a passive attitude is called _____ relaxation. The type of relaxation that encourages people to allow their thoughts to flow without evaluation or censoring is called _____ meditation. Guided imagery asks patients to imagine a _____ image and to concentrate on that image throughout the stressful or painful situation. In general, relaxation is more effective than a _____ and about as effective as biofeedback, which requires expensive equipment.

B. Hypnotic Treatment

Hypnotic procedures have been used for more than 150 years, mostly to help people cope with _____. Although authorities disagree concerning the precise nature of hypnosis, they agree that it includes focused attention and that all hypnosis is _____ - _____. Hypnotic treatment works better than a placebo and provides high levels of relief from a variety of pains, especially for people who are highly _____. However, low suggestible subjects *do not* respond better to hypnosis than to a

_____.

C. Biofeedback

Biofeedback is the process of providing feedback information about the status of _____ systems, which permits people to alter physiological responses that could not have been voluntarily controlled without the feedback. The two most frequently used biofeedback procedures for coping with stress and pain are the _____ (EMG), which measures electrical discharge in muscle fibers, and _____ biofeedback, which uses a thermister to measure skin temperature. Raising skin temperature is the common goal, such as in the treatment of Raynaud's disease, a disorder involving peripheral vascular constriction. Biofeedback is comparable to

_____ training in coping with stress and is better than most

nonmedical treatments for _____ headache.

D. Behavior Modification

Behavior modification techniques are based on the principles of

_____ conditioning, and are used by health psychologists to

help people cope with pain. People in pain usually communicate that fact to

others by complaining, moaning, sighing, limping, rubbing, grimacing, or missing

work, behaviors that often continue because of positive _____

such as attention, sympathy, financial compensation, or relief from work.

Negative reinforcement is the removal of an _____ situation (such

as pain) by taking medication, learning to relax, or some other treatment. With

behavior modification, progress is measured in terms of observable

_____, such as absences from work or level of physical

activity. Behavior modification approaches are at least as effective as cognitive

therapy programs, but their long-term benefits may not be as permanent.

E. Cognitive Therapy

Although cognitive therapy also uses reinforcement, it emphasizes self-

reinforcement more than _____ reinforcers. Cognitive therapy

programs rest on the assumption that when people change their

_____ of an event they can change their emotional and

physiological reaction to that event. Cognitive therapy attempts to get patients

to think differently about their stress or pain experiences and to increase their

_____ -_____ , that is, their confidence that they can perform those behaviors necessary to cope with pain and stress. Donald Meichenbaum and Roy Cameron have developed a strategy for managing stress called stress _____ training, which includes three stages: (1) a reconceptualization stage where patients are encouraged to _____ differently about their stress or pain experiences, (2) an acquisition and _____ of skills stage where patients are taught relaxation and controlled breathing skills, and a (3) _____ -_____ stage where patients apply their coping skills to their daily environment. James Pennebaker and his associates have demonstrated the therapeutic value of expressing _____ emotions and traumatic experiences, a technique called _____. In general, cognitively oriented treatment for stress and pain seems to be at least as effective as either _____ training or _____ modification.

F. Multimodal Approaches

Psychologists sometimes combine several techniques into one multimodal package. This approach is usually _____ the effectiveness of any single procedure, but evaluation of multimodal approaches should consider: (1) whether the extra gain is worth the extra time and _____; (2) that more than a third of patients receiving multimodal strategies are, at the same time, seeking _____ therapies; and (3) the strength of the _____ effect.

Answers

I.   coping
I.A.   social support; half; men; women; networks; medical (health); buffer
I.B.   responsibility
II.A. muscle; imagery; progressive; mediative; mindfulness; peaceful (visual);
       placebo
II.B. pain; self-hypnosis; suggestible; placebo
II.C. physiological (biological); electromyograph; temperature (thermal);
       relaxation; migraine
II.D. operant; reinforcers; aversive; behavior
II.E. environmental (external); interpretation (perception); self-efficacy;
       inoculation; think; rehearsal; follow-through; negative; catharsis;
       relaxation; behavior
II.F. more; expense; nontraditional (alternative); placebo.

Multiple Choice Questions

_____   1. Florence feels emotional concern from her husband, who also
            provides instrumental aid, and communicates love and affection to
            Florence. Thus, Florence receives _____ from her husband.
            a. a social network
            b. social support
            c. unconditional positive regard
            d. agape

_____   2. An absence of social relationships best describes
            a. social network.
            b. social isolation.
            c. sociopathy.
            d. socioeconomic deficiency.

_____   3. The Alameda County study found that
            a. social support is positively linked to heart disease.
            b. social isolation is a risk factor for heart disease for women but
                not for men.
            c. social isolation is an independent risk factor for all-cause
                mortality.
            d. social support is positively related to alcoholism.

_____ 4. The Alameda County study found that
a. marriage benefited men's health more than women's.
b. divorce benefited men's health more than women's.
c. marriage benefited women's health more than men's.
d. marriage helped the health of neither men nor women.

_____ 5. Mildred is a 68-year-old retired teacher. Research suggests that she is most likely to avoid depression if she
a. is married.
b. returns to teaching.
c. performs volunteer work at least twice a week.
d. receives emotional support from a confidant

_____ 6. Which of these personal characteristics is negatively related to receiving social support?
a. hostility
b. succorance
c. friendliness
d. nurturance

_____ 7. If research were to find that institutionalized old people tended to die earlier than old people living at home, we could conclude that
a. old people should not be institutionalized.
b. an absence of social support shortens a person's life span.
c. nursing homes foster feelings of isolation.
d. none of the above

_____ 8. People who believe that their own behavior can affect their health are said to have
a. low self-efficacy.
b. an external locus of control.
c. an internal locus of control.
d. optimistic bias.

_____ 9. Rita, a 70-year-old widow, lives alone except for her two cats. Research suggests that
a. Rita's worry and concern over the health of her cats will have a negative impact on her own health.
b. Rita will make more trips to her doctor than if she did not have any cats.
c. Rita will lose her ability to differentiate between cats and humans.
d. Rita will have somewhat lower blood pressure than if she did not have any pets.

_____ 10. A study by Ellen Langer and Judith Rodin of nursing home residents showed that elderly people were more likely to remain healthy if they
   a. had plants in their rooms.
   b. exercised even small amounts of personal control.
   c. they were able to rearrange their room furniture on a regular basis.
   d. received daily letters from their friends and family.

_____ 11. With this relaxation technique, patients recline in a comfortable chair with no distracting lights or sounds, breathe slowly, and learn to relax different muscle groups:
   a. progressive muscle relaxation.
   b. rational emotive therapy.
   c. hypnosuggestive therapy.
   d. guided imagery.

_____ 12. Health psychologists are most likely to use relaxation training to help people
   a. cope with stress-related problems.
   b. determine their level of pain.
   c. solve marital and other interpersonal problems.
   d. change unhealthy eating habits.

_____ 13. Relaxation training is
   a. most effective in treating imaginary pain.
   b. less effective than biofeedback in treating stress.
   c. more effective than a placebo in relieving pain.
   d. ineffective in relieving pain.

_____ 14. With this relaxation technique, patients focus nonjudgmentally on any thoughts or sensations that occur to them in order to gain insight into how they see the world.
   a. guided imagery
   b. mindfulness meditation
   c. mediative relaxation
   d. rational emotive therapy

_____ 15. Ernest Hilgard and Theodore X. Barber have different opinions on the nature of hypnosis. Their major difference concerns this question:
   a. Does it work?
   b. Is it more effective than a placebo?
   c. Is it an altered state of consciousness?
   d. Does it control pain?

_____ 16. These patients are most likely to benefit from hypnotic treatment when it is used to relieve pain:
   a. children.
   b. people low in suggestibility.
   c. people high in suggestibility.
   d. elderly men.

_____ 17. Health psychologists generally regard the main benefit of hypnotic treatment to be its ability to help people
   a. stop smoking.
   b. cure insomnia.
   c. comply with medical advice.
   d. control pain.

_____ 18. The technique whereby patients learn to control their biological processes such as heart rate or skin temperature is known as
   a. biofeedback.
   b. mindfulness mediation.
   c. mediative relaxation.
   d. guided imagery.

_____ 19. Which technique has been used in an attempt to measure stress, regulate heartbeat, control blood pressure, and reduce pain?
   a. psychoanalysis
   b. biofeedback
   c. rational emotive therapy
   d. cognitive therapy

_____ 20. This type of biofeedback is most likely to be used to control migraine headache:
   a. EMG biofeedback.
   b. temperature biofeedback.
   c. EKG biofeedback.
   d. EEG biofeedback.

_____ 21. This coping strategy relies heavily on operant conditioning principles.
   a. biofeedback
   b. cognitive therapy
   c. behavior modification
   d. guided imagery

_____ 22. Which of these would be an example of a negatively reinforcing situation?
   a. developing a cold after one's spouse gets a cold
   b. achieving pain relief from taking an aspirin
   c. scolding one's child for riding a bicycle without a helmet
   d. getting sick from eating contaminated food.

_____ 23. The notion that certain pain behaviors may be rewarding to the pain patient best fits this technique:
   a. temperature biofeedback.
   b. cognitive therapy.
   c. progressive muscle relaxation.
   d. behavior modification.

_____ 24. Studies on the effectiveness of a pain reduction program are often complicated by this factor:
   a. Spouses unintentionally ignore pain behaviors.
   b. Spouses unintentionally reward pain behaviors.
   c. Single-technique programs are not sufficiently powerful to produce change.
   d. Health psychologists are not adequately trained in pain reduction strategies.

_____ 25. The coping strategy that emphasizes changing the way people think about their stress or pain is
   a. cognitive therapy.
   b. behavior modification.
   c. biofeedback.
   d. hypnosis.

_____ 26. Dennis Turk and Donald Meichenbaum's pain management program is similar to
   a. hypnosis.
   b. stress inoculation.
   c. behavior modification.
   d. biofeedback.

_____ 27. James Pennebaker and his associates found that people who survived traumatic experiences achieved better physical health if they
  a. blocked those experiences from conscious thought.
  b. wrote or talked about those experiences.
  c. were children when they experienced trauma.
  d. were at least 50 years old when they experienced the trauma.

_____ 28. Multimodal approaches to coping with stress and pain are difficult to evaluate because
  a. measures of the dependent variable are unreliable.
  b. they are time consuming.
  c. people receiving a multimodal approach are usually unaware that they are part of an evaluation program.
  d. many people receiving a multimodal approach are receiving nontraditional treatment at the same time

Multiple Choice Answers

1.	b	15.	c
2.	b	16.	c
3.	c	17.	d
4.	a	18.	a
5.	d	19	b
6.	a	20.	b
7.	d	21.	c
8.	c	22.	b
9.	d	23.	d
10.	b	24.	b
11.	a	25.	a
12.	a	26.	b
13.	c	27.	b
14.	b	28.	d

Match the researchers with their research:

1. Wilbert Fordyce

2. Ernest Hilgard

3. James Pennebaker

4. Albert Bandura

5. Neal Miller

6. Ellen Langer and Judith Rodin

7. Donald Meichenbaum and colleagues

8. B. F. Skinner

9. Albert Ellis

a. proposed that irrational beliefs are the basis for many problems.

b. conducted research that formed the basis for behavior modification.

c. proposed that self-efficacy is important in coping with pain and stress.

d. conducted pioneering research on biofeedback.

e. applied behavior modification to the treatment of pain.

f. developed inoculation techniques to deal with stress and pain control.

g. found that hypnosis can be effective for many types of pain control.

h. discovered the importance of personal control for the health of nursing home residents.

i. found that writing about traumatic experiences was therapeutic.

1. e   2. g   3. i   4. c   5. d   6. h   7. f
8. b   9. a

Essay Questions

1. How do the personal resources of social support and personal control affect a person's ability to cope with stress and pain?

2. Which behavioral techniques are effective for coping with pain? Are other techniques better for dealing with stress?

Good points to include in your essay answers:

1. A. Social support is an important factor in health and longevity.
        1. Studies have shown that social support is positively related to low mortality rate.
        2. Emotional support may be more important than other types of support.
            a. Marriage tends to fulfill this need for men, and married men have a health advantage.
            b. Marriage does not profit women's health as much as men's health, but women profit more from social support than men.
    B. Personal control is also important for health.
        1. People who have control over the important aspects of their lives have an internal locus of control, which is generally healthier than an external locus of control.
        2. Studies on nursing home residents by Langer and Rodin demonstrated that even a small degree of personal control can be beneficial to health and lower mortality.

2. A. Techniques that are effective for coping with pain include
        1. Different types of relaxation therapy
            a. Progressive muscle relaxation is effective for tension headache.
            b. Mindfulness meditation can help with several types of chronic pain.
            c. Guided imagery and progressive relaxation can be effective in helping to control nausea associated with cancer chemotherapy.
        2. Hypnotic treatment
            a. Can help hypnotizable people cope successfully with many types of pain but helps less hypnotizable people only as much as a placebo.
            b. Is effective for dental, low back, burn, and childbirth pain.
        3. Different types of biofeedback
            a. The temperature type can be effective in treating migraine headache.
            b. The EMG type can be effective in treating low back pain.
        4. Behavior modification can be effective in decreasing the symptoms associated with a variety of pain syndromes.
        5. Cognitive therapy can be effective with arthritis pain, but it is not as effective as other techniques for migraine headache or low back pain.
    B. The same behavioral techniques can be used for stress, but stress-related problems respond differently.
        1. Hypnotic treatment and behavior modification are used for pain control more than stress management.
        2. Several types of relaxation are effective for coping with anxiety, and relaxation and have some positive effect on hypertension.
        3. Biofeedback is no more effective than relaxation for stress problems.
        4. The cognitive therapy techniques of stress inoculation and writing about traumatic events are effective in dealing with stress and anxiety.

Let's Get Personal—
What Are Your Coping Resources?

Everyone experiences stress, but all people are not equally vulnerable to the negative effects of stress. Personal resources for coping affect vulnerability, and these resources include social support and techniques for coping. How extensive are your resources?

These analyses of your social support and typical coping strategies should allow you to pinpoint areas in which you can function more effectively. Perhaps you need to build a more extensive or a more reliable social support network, or perhaps you need to develop a wider variety of coping strategies that are appropriate to the stresses you experience.

When I have a personal or emotional problem, these people will help me—

When I have a problem related to my work or school, these people will help me—

When I have a financial problem, these people will help me—

How many people form your social support network?

Do they respond when you ask, or do they anticipate your needs?

What relationship do these people have to you—family or friends?

In which areas do you have the best social support?

In which areas might your social support network be lacking?

When I experience a personal of emotional problem, I typically (check as many as apply)

- ☐ Turn to friends for emotional support.

- ☐ Turn to family for emotional support.

- ☐ Analyze what actions to take to alleviate the problem.

- ☐ Try not to think about it too much.

- ☐ Do something to take my mind off my problems.

When I experience a work- or school-related problem, I typically (check as many as apply)

- ☐ Turn to friends for emotional support.

- ☐ Turn to family for emotional support.

- ☐ Analyze what actions to take to alleviate the problem.

- ☐ Try not to think about it too much.

- ☐ Do something to take my mind off my problems.

When I experience financial problems, I typically (check as many as apply)

- ☐ Turn to friends for emotional support.

- ☐ Turn to family for emotional support.

- ☐ Analyze what actions to take to alleviate the problem.

- ☐ Try not to think about it too much.

- ☐ Do something to take my mind off my problems.

Do you manage stress by active problem solving, by passive avoidance, or do you choose active coping for some types of stressors and passive avoidance for other stressors? If you try to avoid thinking about the problem or if you do something to take your mind off your problems, do you increase your health risks by drinking, taking drugs, or engage in other risky behaviors as ways to avoid your problems?

CHAPTER 9
Identifying Behavioral Factors in Cardiovascular Disease

Fill in the Rest of the Story

I. The Cardiovascular System

The cardiovascular system, consisting of the heart and blood vessels,

transports _____ throughout the body, providing a means of

delivering oxygen and nutrients and also removing wastes from cells.

Oxygenated blood is carried from the heart by vessels called

_____ , and blood that has been released of its oxygen is

returned to the heart by the _____.

A. The Coronary Arteries

Blood is delivered to the myocardium (the _____ muscle) by the

_____ arteries. Any damage to the coronary arteries can be

hazardous. The formation of atheromatous plaque restricts the flow of blood to

the myocardium, resulting in occlusion of the arteries is called

_____. Loss of elasticity or hardening of the arteries is called

_____.

B. Coronary Artery Disease

Coronary heart disease results from the buildup of _____ in the

coronary arteries and may result in restriction of blood flow to the heart, a

135

condition known as _____. This restriction may produce chest

pain and difficulty in breathing and is called _____

_____. Myocardial infarction (often called _____

_____) is a much more serious coronary heart disease.

C. Stroke

When atherosclerosis and arteriosclerosis affect the arteries that deliver

blood to the _____, stroke becomes increasingly possible. A

restriction of the _____ supply to the brain or to part of the brain

results in the death of neurons and the loss of function performed by those

neurons.

D. Blood Pressure

Blood pressure is measured by two numbers: the pressure exerted by

ventricular contractions, called _____ pressure, and the

pressure between contractions, called _____ pressure.

Hypertension, or _____ blood pressure, may result from several

different causes, but the most common is _____ hypertension,

which has no identifiable cause but is a risk factor for cardiovascular disease.

Secondary hypertension is much less common and results from other disease

processes.

II. Measures of Cardiovascular Function

The most common measurement of cardiovascular function is

_____ _____, but this measure does not reveal important factors in cardiac functioning, such as the regularity of the heartbeat or the amount of blood reaching the myocardium.

A. Measurements of Electrical Activity in the Heart

A measure of the electrical activity of the heart taken either while a person is at rest or exercising is an _____, or ECG. An exercise ECG is called a _____ test and will reveal about 50% of CVD cases, compared to about _____ percent detection rate by resting ECG.

B. Angiography

The procedure that involves passing a catheter into the circulatory system to inject dye into the heart and then to X-ray the heart is called

_____. The procedure that involves cardiac catheterization and the flattening of atherosclerotic deposits in order to improve circulation is known as _____.

III. The Changing Rates of Cardiovascular Disease

During the past 35 years, deaths from heart attack and stroke in the United States have declined sharply. Nevertheless, cardiovascular disease (heart disease and stroke) remains the leading cause of death. accounting for almost _____ percent of all deaths.

A. Reasons for the Decline in Death Rates

The decline in CVD deaths has been due mostly to two factors: a change in

_____ of people in the United States, and improved medical care for cardiac patients. Evidence that lifestyle changes play an important role in the decreasing death rates from CVD is found in research showing a decline in _____ heart attack. Three lifestyle changes that may have contributed to this decline are: better diet, increased levels of physical activity, and lower rates of _____.

B. Heart Disease Mortality throughout the World

Countries other than the United States have also experienced lower CVD death rates. Studies from Finland, New Zealand, and Australia show that changes in lifestyle account for at least _____ percent of the drop in CVD mortality.

IV. Risk Factors in Cardiovascular Disease

Much information about risk factors for cardiovascular disease has come from one study—the _____ Heart Study, begun in 1948. Results of this and other epidemiological studies have brought the concept of risk factor into popular usage. Risk factors do not prove _____ but simply provide information concerning which conditions are _associated_ with a particular disease.

A. Inherent Risk Factors

Inherent risk factors result from _____ or physical conditions that cannot be changed through modification of lifestyle. Inherent risk factors for cardiovascular disease include: juvenile-onset diabetes, age, family history of

cardiovascular disease, ethnic background (_____ Americans

are at increased risk), and perhaps gender; _____ have a greater risk

than _____ for CVD mortality, especially before age 60.

B. Physiological Conditions

The best predictor of CVD is _____, or high blood pressure.

Another important physiological risk is serum _____,

which circulates in the blood in several different forms of lipoprotein.

_____-density lipoprotein protects against cardiovascular disease,

whereas _____-density lipoprotein contributes to the disease. The

ratio of total cholesterol to _____ - _____

_____ cholesterol seems to be a better predictor of heart disease

than total cholesterol.   Low-density lipoprotein is difficult to reduce, but

eliminating _____ fats (red meats, whole milk, and eggs) from

one's diet is effective for most people. Not all people need to worry about high

cholesterol, because _____ people are at lower risk than younger

people.

C. Behavioral Factors

The two leading behavioral risk factors for cardiovascular disease are diet

and _____.   Diets high in saturated fat are

_____ related to heart disease, whereas those low in saturated fat protect against heart disease. Vitamin E, beta carotene, selenium, and riboflavin have been identified as _____ that provide some protection against CVD. Diets high in _____ tend to be low in fat and to offer additional protection against heart disease.

D. Psychosocial Factors

Psychosocial factors related to CVD include anxiety, educational level, income level, marriage, social support, the _____ _____ behavior pattern, and hostility. The relationship between anxiety and heart disease is stronger for _____ than it is for _____. Low educational level and low income are both _____ related to heart disease. In addition, people with higher income levels are more likely than those at low income levels to _____ coronary disease, which suggests that being able to afford good medical care may prolong one's life. For most people, being single and having little _____ _____ increases the risk of CVD. During the past 2 or 3 decades, researchers have looked to personality variables and behavior patterns as possible risks for CVD. The best known of these variables is the Type A _____ _____, which includes competitiveness, concern with numbers, the acquisition of objects, an exaggerated sense of time urgency, and _____. Lately, however, support for the Type A behavior has not been strong. Of all the original components of the Type A behavior pattern, the one most related to heart disease was hostility, especially _____ hostility. The relationship of this

component and CHD may be mediated through _____, the

tendency to react strongly to stressful or emotional situations. Because hostility

relates to gender, ethnicity, educational level, and socioeconomic status, and other

factors that are risk factors for CHD, some researchers have questioned whether

hostility is an _____ risk. Some of these researchers have

narrowed their investigations to a specific component of hostility, namely

_____. Even more specifically, the _____ of

anger may be more toxic than the experience of anger. Although expressing

anger puts people at increased risk, research indicates that _____

anger is also a risk for heart disease.

V. Modifying Risk Factors for Cardiovascular Disease

Changing risky behaviors and lifestyles are difficult for several reasons,

including the tendency of many people to have an optimistic bias.

A. Reducing Hypertension

One difficulty in reducing high blood pressure is that many hypertensive

people are _____ of their condition. Stress management

programs, weight loss, sodium restriction, exercise, and reduced consumption of

alcohol are several nonpharmacological strategies for reducing hypertension.

B. Lowering Serum Cholesterol

Serum cholesterol is also resistant to changes through behavioral means, but exercise and _____ are two methods that have had some success.

C. Modifying Psychosocial Risk Factors

Several interventions have been designed to modify cynical hostility and

anger. Redford Williams has outlined a 12-step program designed to help people

to reduce cynical _____ by learning to relax and to trust others.

Aron Seigman has trained people to be aware of their toxic anger and to

_____ anger with a calm, slow speech pattern.

Answers

I.	blood; arteries; veins
I.A.	heart; coronary; atherosclerosis; arteriosclerosis
I.B.	plaque; ischemia; angina pectoris; heart attack
I.C.	brain; blood (oxygen)
I.D.	systolic; diastolic; high; essential
II.	blood pressure
II.A.	electrocardiogram; stress; 25,
II.B.	angiography; angioplasty
III.	40
III.A.	lifestyle; first; smoking
III.B.	50
IV.	Framingham; causation
IV.A.	genetic; African; men; women
IV.B.	hypertension; cholesterol; High; low; high-density lipoprotein; saturated; older
IV.C.	smoking; positively; antioxidants; fiber
IV.D.	Type A; men; women; positively; survive; social support; behavior pattern; hostility; cynical; hyperreactivity (reactivity); independent; anger; suppressed
V.A.	unaware
V.B.	diet
V.C.	hostility; express

Multiple Choice Questions

_____ 1. Which one of these persons has the LOWEST risk for heart disease?
   a. a 45-year-old man who openly and loudly expresses anger to others
   b. a 45-year-old man who suppresses his anger to avoid conflict
   c. a 75-year-old European American woman living alone
   d. a 35-year-old European American woman living alone
   e. a 50-year-old African American married man.

_____ 2. The circulation of blood
   a. transports carbon dioxide to body cells.
   b. transports oxygen to body cells.
   c. removes carbon dioxide from body cells.
   d. both b and c

_____ 3. Blood is furnished to the heart by way of
   a. coronary veins.
   b. coronary arteries.
   c. arterioles.
   d. anterior venules.

_____ 4. The technical name for heart attack is
   a. arrhythmia.
   b. angina pectoris.
   c. atherosclerosis
   d. myocardial infarction.

_____ 5. Atherosclerosis is
   a. a narrowing of the arteries.
   b. the loss of elasticity of the arteries.
   c. another name for heart attack.
   d. characterized by a crushing pain in the chest.

_____ 6. Arteriosclerosis is
   a. a narrowing of the arteries.
   b. the loss of elasticity of the arteries.
   c. another name for heart attack.
   d. characterized by a crushing pain in the chest.

_____ 7. After feeling a crushing pain in the chest and difficulty in breathing, Roscoe went to a cardiologist who found no damage to Roscoe's myocardium. Roscoe was probably diagnosed as having
a. a heart attack.
b. a myocardial infarction.
c. a stroke.
d. angina pectoris.

_____ 8. Restriction of blood flow to the brain results in
a. a stroke.
b. an embolism.
c. angina pectoris.
d. a myocardial infarction.

_____ 9. Which of these blood pressure readings would be normal for an adult?
a. systolic pressure of 130; diastolic pressure of 70
b. diastolic pressure of 130; systolic pressure of 70
c. diastolic pressure of 150; systolic pressure of 110
d. systolic pressure of 150; diastolic pressure of 110

_____ 10. Which of these would be the best predictor of cardiovascular disease?
a. Type A behavior pattern
b. high levels of high-density lipoprotein
c. being 15 to 20 pounds overweight
d. high blood pressure

_____ 11. A stress test is used to measure
a. the number of stressful life events a person has experienced during the past year.
b. the intensity of stressful life events a person has experienced during the past year.
c. the heart's electrical activity during exercise.
d. the heart's electrical activity during sleep.

_____ 12. Estel has undergone a procedure in which a dye was injected into her heart to provide her doctors with a view of her coronary arteries through X-ray. This procedure is called
a. a stress test.
b. cardiac angiography.
c. angioplasty.
d. an electrocardiogram.

_____ 13. During the past 40 years, the death rate from cardiovascular disease in the United States has
  a. dropped steadily.
  b. remained about the same.
  c. increased slightly.
  d. increased sharply.

_____ 14. The decline in the rate of first heart attacks strongly suggests that the overall drop in cardiovascular mortality
  a. is a temporary phenomenon.
  b. is due to improved medical procedures.
  c. results at least partially from changes in lifestyle.
  d. results from lower rates of compliance.

_____ 15. Which of these is most clearly an inherent risk factor for cardiovascular disease?
  a. gender
  b. a high fat diet
  c. hostility
  d. hypertension

_____ 16. A risk factor for heart disease is
  a. any known cause of heart disease.
  b. any condition that predicts heart disease.
  c. any condition that results from heart disease.
  d. any condition that results in a decline in rate of heart disease.

_____ 17. Which of these ethnic groups has the highest rates of cardiovascular mortality?
  a. African Americans
  b. Asian Americans
  c. European Americans
  d. Hispanic Americans

_____ 18. The strongest inherent risk factor for cardiovascular disease is
  a. family history.
  b. smoking.
  c. advancing age.
  d. gender.

_____ 19. Although high total cholesterol is positively related to cardiovascular disease,
    a. low-density lipoprotein is negatively related to CVD.
    b. high-density lipoprotein is negatively related to CVD.
    c. low-density lipoprotein has a curvilinear relationship with CVD.
    d. high-density lipoprotein has a curvilinear relationship with CVD.

_____ 20. HDL can be raised through
    a. exercise.
    d. decreased consumption of alcohol.
    c. quitting smoking.
    d. a diet high in saturated fats.

_____ 21. Total cholesterol
    a. is a better predictor of heart disease than the ratio of total cholesterol to HDL.
    b. does not seem to be a risk factor for heart disease among elderly people.
    c. does not seem to be a risk factor for heart disease among children.
    d. both a and b

_____ 22. Low levels of total cholesterol are associated with increased risk of
    a. heart attack.
    b. stroke.
    c. diabetes.
    d. suicide.

_____ 23. Smoking, a known risk factor for lung cancer,
    a. is not a risk factor for heart disease.
    b. is a risk factor for heart disease for men but not for women.
    c. is a risk factor for heart disease for women but not for men.
    d. is a strong risk for heart disease for both men and women.

_____ 24. Celina, a manager of a retail clothing store, wants to reduce her risk for cardiovascular disease. She is 28 years old, about 15 pounds over her ideal weight, smokes a pack of cigarettes a day, drinks moderately, and has no family history of heart disease. Celina's best course of action would be to
   a. lose 20 pounds.
   b. stop smoking.
   c. stop drinking alcohol.
   d. quit her job.
   e. stop eating foods cooked in polyunsaturated fats.

_____ 25. Although obesity may not be an independent risk factor for cardiovascular disease, it is often related to
   a. hypertension.
   b. a sedentary life style.
   c. high cholesterol levels.
   d. all of the above

_____ 26. Anxiety is
   a. positively related to nonfatal heart attack.
   b. negatively related to nonfatal heart attack.
   c. positively related to fatal heart attack.
   d. negatively related to fatal heart attack.

_____ 27. This component of the original Type A behavior pattern has received the most support as a risk factor for heart disease:
   a. state anxiety.
   b. a sense of time urgency.
   c. hostility.
   d. a strong sense of competition.

_____ 28. Researchers have found that _____ is the toxic component of hostility.
   a. repressed hostility
   b. repressed anxiety
   c. expressed anger
   d. interpersonal trust

_____ 29. People at risk for heart disease should
   a. openly and loudly express their anger.
   b. remain calm and suppress their anger.
   c. express their anger in a soft, slow manner.
   d. avoid any situation that might arouse their anger.

Multiple Choice Answers

1.	d	16.	b
2.	d	17.	a
3.	b	18.	c
4.	d	19.	b
5.	a	20.	a
6.	b	21.	b
7.	d	22.	d
8.	a	23.	d
9.	a	24.	b
10.	d	25.	d
11.	c	26.	c
12.	b	27.	c
13.	a	28.	c
14.	c	29.	c
15.	a		

Evolution of the Type A Concept

Research on the toxic components of the Type A behavior pattern has evolved from the global pattern to more specific elements. Fill in the missing components in the following figure, arranging your answers so that the last item is the one that prompted further research.

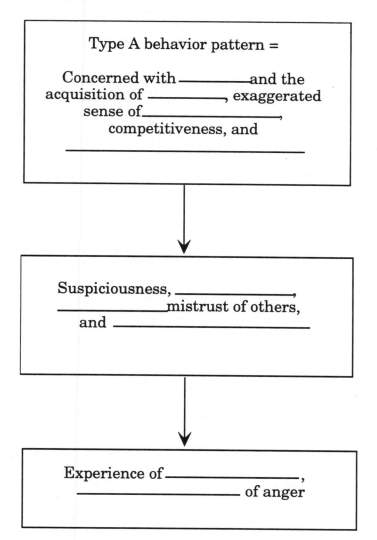

Essay Questions

1. Trace the development of the Type A behavior pattern to its current status.

2. Clint is a 35-year-old man who wants to lower his risk of developing cardiovascular disease. Give him some advice.

Good points to include in your essay answers:

1. A. The concept of the Type A behavior pattern
    1. Originated by cardiologists Friedman and Rosenman.
    2. Included a pattern of behavior characteristic of coronary patients, including time pressure, competition, concern with money, impatience, and hostility.
    B. Support for the Type A concept came from the Western Collaborative Group Study, which found that men classified as Type A were twice as likely as Type B men to develop coronary heart disease.
    C. Other research has failed to support the global Type A behavior pattern as a risk for CVD, but research turned to hostility and anger as possible toxic components.
    D. Hostility is a better predictor of heart disease than is the Type A behavior pattern but may not be an independent risk factor.
    E. Anger has become the current topic of research interest concerning cardiovascular risk, and both suppressed and expressed anger are risk, but expressed anger is the greater risk.

2. A. Clint's risks depend on his inherent risk factors as well as his behaviors and habits, but he can lower his risks by changing his behavior.
    B. Clint should know his blood pressure and try to either keep his blood pressure in the normal range or bring his hypertension back toward normal.
    1. Losing weight can lower blood pressure for people who are overweight.
    2. Complying to blood pressure medication can be important.
    C. Clint should not smoke.
    D. Clint should eat a diet low in fat and high in fiber in an attempt to maintain or attain serum cholesterol level below 200.
    1. If his cholesterol level is high, he may not be able to lower it through diet alone.
    2. He should be concerned about the ratio of total cholesterol to high-density lipoprotein (HDL), striving for a high HDL count.
    E. Clint should express any anger in with a slow, soft voice and try to avoid any expression of cynical hostility.

Let's Get Personal—
Will Cardiovascular Disease Happen to You?

Do you believe that you will develop cardiovascular disease? Recall that almost 40% of deaths in the United States are due to cardiovascular disease, so you are probably more likely to develop cardiovascular disease (CVD) than any other life-threatening disease. If you are a college student in your 20s, this possibility may seem very remote because cardiovascular disease is associated with middle-aged and elderly adults. The processes that result in CVD, however, begin during youth, and you may be building your risks right now.

What risk factors for CVD do you have? Answering the following questions will help you understand how this family of diseases can affect you.

Do you know your blood pressure, and is it in the normal range?

Do you eat a high-fat diet—that is, a diet in which more than 30% of calories come from fat?

Do you eat five or more servings of fruits and vegetables per day?

What is your total cholesterol level?

Is your high-density lipoprotein ratio in the desirable range?

Do you smoke?

Do you follow a regular exercise program that gives you aerobic benefits?

Do many things anger you, and do you interpret the action of others as intentionally annoying?

Do you express your anger in ways that present cardiovascular risks, such a yelling?

When you are angry, do you try to suppress your anger rather than expressing it?

Do you use stimulant drugs such as amphetamines or cocaine?

Although few young people die of cardiovascular disease, many have habits that will lead to CVD. If you believe that heart disease will not happen to you, the odds may not be in your favor.

CHAPTER 10
Identifying Behavioral Factors in Cancer

Fill in the Rest of the Story

I. Cancer and Its Changing Mortality Rates

Cancer is an ancient disease, but it was not well understood until physicians began to use microscopes and dissection.

A. What Is Cancer?

Different cancer cells share a common characteristic; namely, the presence of

_____ tissue, or cells that have nearly unlimited growth and that rob the host of nutrients. Neoplastic cells can be either _____ or malignant. Malignant tumors are the more dangerous because they

_____; that is, they invade and destroy surrounding tissue. Malignant growths are divided into four main groups: carcinomas, or cancerous cells of the skin, stomach lining, and mucous membranes;

_____, or cancerous cells of the connective tissue, such as bones, muscles, and cartilage; leukemias, or cancers that originate in the

_____ ; and _____, cancer of the lymphatic system.

B. The Changing Mortality Rates from Cancer

Cancer is the second leading cause of death in the United States, but during the past 4 or 5 years, mortality rates from cancer have begun to decline. Most

cancer deaths in the United States are associated with _____

and personal behavior, with cigarette smoking and _____ being

the two leading psychosocial risk factors.

II. Behavioral Risk Factors for Cancer

Although heredity plays a role in the development of cancer, about two-

thirds of all cancer deaths in the United States are associated with

_____ and unwise eating habits.

A. Smoking

Cigarette smokers have at least _____ the risk of death

compared to nonsmokers and about 9 to 10 times the risk of death from

_____ cancer. This excess risk is the largest risk for any

behavior and a major cause of death. In addition, the more cigarettes a person

smokes the greater the chances of developing cancer; that is, the risk is

_____ _____. Many smokers believe that the

negative effects of smoking affect others but not themselves; that is, they possess

an _____ _____ that tends to perpetuate their

risky behavior. When smoking is combined with exposure to air pollution and

building materials such as asbestos, the risk of lung cancer becomes more than

additive—it becomes _____. In general, the risk of lung

cancer from smoking cigars and pipes is _____ than the risk from

smoking cigarettes.

B. Diet

Perhaps 60% of all cancer in _____ and _____ percent of all cancer in men can be linked to diet, with cancers of the breast, stomach, uterus, endometrium, rectum, colon, kidneys, small intestine, pancreas, liver, ovaries, bladder, prostate, mouth, pharynx, thyroid, and esophagus all having a dietary link. In general, the same foods that have been linked to _____ disease are also associated with cancer. These include beef, pork, dairy products, and others foods with heavy concentrations of _____ fat.Other foods, including vitamin supplements, have been promoted as protection against cancer. Consumption of dietary _____ from _____ and fruits is associated with lower rates of colon and _____ cancers.

C. Alcohol

Alcohol is probably a _____ risk factor for cancer, but it may have a synergistic effect when combined with _____ _____, placing some heavy drinkers at a much greater risk of cancer of the larynx.

D. Physical Activity

Physical activity may offer some protection against cancer. Moderate exercise is related to lower rates of colon and _____ cancers in men and colon and _____ cancer in women.

E. Ultraviolet Light

The most common form of cancer in the United States is _____ cancer, but death rates from this cancer are relatively low. However, one form of skin cancer—malignant _____—has a high death rate. North Americans who live in sunny climates are especially vulnerable to skin cancer if they are _____-skinned.

F. Sexual Behavior

Sexual behavior plays a role in cancers that result from AIDS, such as _____ sarcoma and non-Hodgkin's _____. For women, early age at first _____ and a large number of _____ _____ increase the risks for cancer of the cervix, vagina, and ovaries. Conversely, early _____ and childbirth may offer some protection against breast cancer.

III. Risk Factors Beyond Personal Control

Besides behavioral factors, environmental and inherent conditions can contribute to the development of cancer.

A. Environmental Risk Factors

Environmental factors include exposure to radiation, asbestos, pesticides, and other chemicals. These environmental risks are quite small and difficult to estimate. Some evidence suggests that long-time exposure to radiation may increase cancer risks for people who work in a

_____ power plant, but not for people who work with X-rays.

B. Inherent Risk Factors for Cancer

Inherent risk factors for cancer include family history, ethnic

background, and _____. Family history can be an important

factor in predicting _____ cancer in women. Having a mother or

sister with early breast cancer doubles or triples a woman's risk for this disease.

Compared with European Americans, _____ Americans have a

40% to 50% greater incidence and mortality from cancer, and much of this

increased risk is probably related to _____ status.

As with heart disease, the greatest risk factor for cancer is advancing

_____; the older people become the greater their chances of dying of

cancer.

IV. Psychological Risk Factors for Cancer

Psychological conditions present only a weak risk for cancer, but they can

interact with behavioral and inherent risks to increase one's chances for cancer.

Two psychological risks are depression and suppression of

_____ .

A. Suppression of Emotion

The inability to express emotions, such as hostility and

_____ may relate positively to some cancers. "Acting out" and

openly displaying emotions may _____ against cancer

B. Depression

Evidence for a relationship between depression and the subsequent development of cancer is not strong. Depression is more strongly related to the _____ of cancer than to its development.

V. Psychosocial Factors and Survival of Cancer Patients

Psychosocial factors not only relate to the development of cancer, but they also predict _____ time for people with terminal cancer. Rejection of the cancer diagnosis tends to _____ life expectancy for cancer patients. Being married, receiving _____ support, and adopting a "fighting spirit" also seem to increase survival time. In addition, receiving psychotherapy that allows expression of strong _____ may add months to the survival time of cancer patients.

Answers

I.A   neoplastic; benign; metastasize; sarcomas; blood; lymphomas
I.B.   lifestyle; diet
II.   smoking (cigarettes)
II.A.   double (twice); lung; dose related; optimistic bias; synergistic; less (lower)
II.B.   women; 40; heart (cardiovascular); saturated (animal); fiber; vegetables; rectal
II.C.   weak (minor); cigarette smoking
II.D.   prostate; breast
II.E.   skin; melanoma; light (fair)
II.F.   Kaposi's; lymphoma; intercourse; sex partners; pregnancy
III.A. nuclear
III.B. age; breast; African; socioeconomic; age
IV.   emotion
IV.A.   anger (rage); protect
IV.B.   advancement (spread)
V.   survival; increase; social; emotions

Multiple Choice Questions

_____ 1. A common side effect of chemotherapy is
a. weight gain.
b. impaired vision.
c. depression.
d. loss of hair.

_____ 2. Which of these is the strongest risk factor for cancer?
a. a high fiber diet
b. environmental chemicals.
c. a low fiber diet high in saturated fat.
d. alcohol

_____ 3. Unlike benign tumors, malignant tumors
a. attack only tissue cells.
b. can metastasize.
c. grow more slowly.
d. cannot metastasize.

_____ 4. Currently, cancer mortality is increasing most sharply for
a. lung cancer among men.
b. lung cancer among women.
c. stomach cancer.
d. breast cancer.

_____ 5. The type of cancer that accounts for the greatest number of malignancies is
a. sarcomas.
b. leukemias.
c. lymphomas.
d. carcinomas.

_____ 6. Diet has been identified as a strong risk factor for
a. cancer but not heart disease.
b. heart disease but not cancer.
c. neither heart disease nor cancer.
d. both heart disease and cancer.

_____ 7. Which of these factors has contributed most to cancer death rates in the United States during the past 50 years?
   a. pesticides
   b. carcinogens in the drinking water
   c. sexual practices
   d. cigarette smoking

_____ 8. This cancer kills more women in the United States than any other:
   a. lung cancer.
   b. breast cancer.
   c. stomach cancer.
   d. cancer of the uterus.

_____ 9. This cancer kills more men in the United States than any other:
   a. lung cancer.
   b. prostrate cancer.
   c. stomach cancer.
   d. colon cancer.

_____ 10. Except for _____ cancer, total death rates from cancer have declined during the past 4 or 5 years.
   a. lung
   b. colon
   c. rectal
   d. bone

_____ 11. Cancer death rates are highest for
   a. children below age 12.
   b. adolescents and young adults.
   c. middle-aged adults.
   d. elderly people.

_____ 12. Compared with cigarette smokers, people who smoke only pipes
   a. have the same risk for cancer.
   b. have about two thirds the risk for cancer.
   c. have about one third the risk for cancer.
   d. have almost no risk for cancer.

_____ 13. From 1993 to 1997, cancer death rates in the United States
   a. increased sharply for both men and women.
   b. increased sharply for men but remained about the same for women.
   c. increased sharply for women but remained about the same for men.
   d. declined slightly.

_____ 14. Which of these factors account for the most total deaths from cancer in the United States?
  a. alcohol
  b. diet
  c. ultraviolet light
  d. sexual practices

_____ 15. Sandy, a 20-year-old college student, wants to do whatever is possible to avoid cancer. Which diet offers her the best protection against cancer?
  a. "natural" foods with no preservatives
  b. salt-cured foods
  c. a diet high in grains, fruits, and vegetables
  d. a high protein diet, featuring meat and dairy products

_____ 16. Research indicates that dietary fiber
  a. offers some protection against cancer of the colon and rectum.
  b. promotes lung and breast cancer.
  c. promotes the growth of tumors.
  d. has a positive relationship with lymphoma.

_____ 17. The ingredient in pizza that may offer some protection against cancer is (are)
  a. the tomato sauce.
  b. the mushrooms.
  c. the anchovies.
  d. the cheese

_____ 18. Alcohol
  a. is not a risk factor for cancer.
  b. is a strong risk factor for cancer.
  c. is generally a strong risk factor for cancer, but it effects are limited to colon cancer.
  d. is generally a weak risk factor for cancer, but it can have a synergistic effect with smoking that increases people's risk of laryngeal cancer.

_____ 19. This cancer is the most frequent type of cancer in the United States, but it is often not fatal:
  a. leukemia.
  b. skin cancer.
  c. rectal cancer.
  d. Kaposi's sarcoma.

_____ 20. A "prudent" pattern of eating may offer some protection against colon cancer. Such a diet includes mostly
    a. red meat and processed meat.
    b. fruits, vegetables, and some fish.
    c. sugars.
    d. refined grains.

_____ 21. The incidence of Kaposi's sarcoma and non-Hodgkin's lymphoma increased during the 1980s due to
    a. increased alcohol consumption.
    b. exposure to the sun.
    c. HIV infection and AIDS.
    d. increased environmental pollutants.

_____ 22. Which of these factors is positively related to cancer of the cervix?
    a. late age at first intercourse
    b. high socioeconomic status
    c. having many sex partners
    d. having first child late in life

_____ 23. Which of these psychosocial factors is most strongly related to the development of cancer?
    a. stressful life events
    b. suppression of emotions
    c. extraversion
    d. Type A behavior pattern
    e. depression

_____ 24. Which personality type seems to be most susceptible to cancer?
    a. people who overtly and aggressively express their feelings
    b. people who have a hopeless and helpless attitude
    c. depressed people
    c. psychologically autonomous people

_____ 25. Which of these factors has the strongest relationship to cancer?
    a. living near a nuclear power plant
    b. being exposed to pesticides as a child
    c. age
    d. gender

_____ 26. Cancer patients who participated in group therapy that included an opportunity to receive emotional support and express negative emotions
   a. had a better emotional adjustment than other patients but had similar survival times.
   b. had a better emotional adjustment and longer survival time than other cancer patients.
   c. tended to be more poorly adjusted and had poorer immune system function than other patients.
   d. had more emotional conflicts with their families than other cancer patients.

_____ 27. People who do not smoke, eat a high-fiber diet, and avoid sun exposure
   a. are still likely to get cancer.
   b. decrease their risk of getting cancer.
   c. do not make significant changes in their cancer risk.
   d. will be so miserable that they will wish they had gotten cancer.

Multiple Choice Answers

1.	d		15.	c
2.	c		16.	a
3.	b		17.	a
4.	b		18.	d
5.	d		19.	b
6.	d		20.	b
7.	d		21.	c
8.	a		22.	c
9.	a		23.	b
10.	a		24.	b
11.	d		25.	c
12.	c		26.	b
13.	d		27.	b
14.	b			

Changes in Cancer Rates

The following figures represent changes in several of the leading causes of cancer deaths over the past 70 years. Label the types of cancer deaths for men and for women.

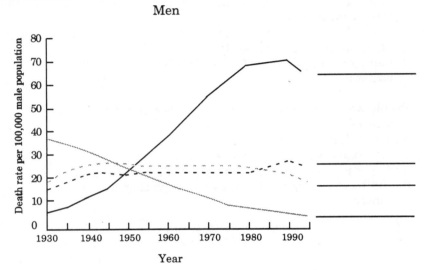

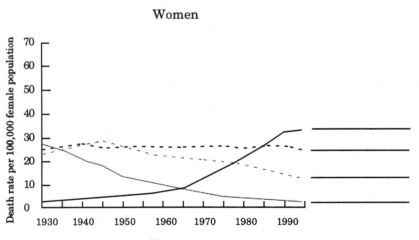

Essay Questions

1. Garland is a smoker who believes that air pollution is the major cause of lung cancer. Is his belief accurate, and what is probably responsible for his attitude?

2.   Alice wants to protect herself against cancer. What should she do?

Good points to include in your essay answers:

1. A. Garland's belief is inaccurate. The threat from air pollution is minor in comparison with that from smoking.
       1. Estimates for increases in the risk for lung cancer among smokers varies from about 9 times to 50 times that for nonsmokers.
       2. This link is the strongest for any behavior-illness pairing.
    B. Like Garland, smokers tend to have a perceived risk that is not as strong as the actual risk.
       1. This perception is the result of optimistic bias that makes smokers believe that the negative consequences of smoking will not happen to them.
       2. One study showed that almost half of smokers said that no strong evidence has demonstrated that smoking causes cancer, and over 40% said that something else causes cancer.
       3. People who engage in risky behaviors have trouble acknowledging that their behavior places them at risk.

2. A. Alice probably cannot completely protect herself against cancer.
       1. Some cancers have a hereditary component.
       2. Many environmental factors relate to the development of cancer, and avoiding all would be impossible.
    B. Alice can lower her risk in several ways.
       1. She should not smoke or use any other form of tobacco.
       2. She should avoid a high-fat diet and concentrate on increasing her intake of fruits, vegetables, and grains.
       3. She should avoid excessive drinking, especially in combination with smoking.
       4. She should participate in physical exercise.
       5. She should avoid sun exposure and should not try to develop a tan.
       6. She should avoid risky sexual behaviors, but she should keep in mind that
          a. Early intercourse raises the risk for reproductive cancers.
          b. Early pregnancy decreases the risk for breast cancer.
       7. She should try to develop healthy strategies for expressing emotion and avoid a helpless and hopeless attitude toward life events.

Let's Get Personal—
Are You Increasing Your Risk?

Cancer is complex, consisting of several different types of malignancies that affect a variety of body sites. The major risk factors for cancer are behaviors, and you may have habits that increase your risk. In addition, you may be at risk for cancer as a result of hereditary or environmental factors beyond your control. Although the research indicates that personal behaviors provide the biggest risks, people have trouble accepting that they are behaving in ways that are harmful.

To understand how your behavior may be raising your risk for cancer, choose a type of cancer for which your risk is elevated. If you do not know of any type for which you have an elevated risk, you may determine your risk by completing one of the brief cancer screenings offered by the American Cancer Society. Once you have chosen a type of cancer, research the risk factors that increase the chances of developing it, beginning with the information in your textbook. When you have discovered the risks, divide them into behavioral versus hereditary and environmental. Which type of risk factors raise the relative risk more? If the type of cancer you have researched is like most types, the behavioral risks are bigger, and you may be doing things that raise your risk.

Type of cancer—

How high is your risk compared to other people your age?

What are the behaviors that elevate the risk for this type of cancer?

What are the environmental and hereditary factors that elevate the risk?

Which type of factor increases the risk more dramatically—behavioral or environmental/hereditary?

How can you lower your risk?

CHAPTER 11
Living with Chronic Illness

Fill in the Rest of the Story

I. The Impact of Chronic Illness

The diagnosis of a _____ illness may present a crisis, but adjustment to the illness may change the way patients see themselves, produce financial strain, and disrupt established patterns of personal and social behaviors.

A. Impact on the Patient

Chronically ill patients are more likely to survive and to get well if they have strong _____ _____ from friends and family members. Support groups can be valuable for people with chronic illness, providing information as well as emotional support. Health psychologists can also provide assistance in helping chronically ill people cope with negative emotions and gain a sense of _____ over their condition.

B Impact on the Family

For chronically ill children, the disease may become an important aspect in their _____ formation and may limit their activities and mobility. Patents of sick children often experience marital discord and financial distress, and many join support groups to cope with these problems.

II. Following a Cardiac Rehabilitation Program

An increasing number of heart attack victims are surviving and follow a cardiac rehabilitation program that includes medication, smoking cessation, regular _____, and a low-fat, low-salt diet. Heart attack patients who participate in cardiac rehabilitation programs have _____ death rates than those who do not.

A. Lifestyle Changes

If heart patients wish to reduce their chances of another heart attack, they must make lifestyle changes, including a low-fat diet, _____ cessation, _____ exercise, and stress reduction.

B. Psychological Reactions After Heart Disease

Many cardiac patients suffer deep anxiety, sleep disturbance, and concern about a second heart attack, but the most common psychological reaction is _____. A significant number of cardiac patients suffer from psychological disorders, such as delusions and paranoia. Also, the patient's spouse often feels depressed and angry.

C. Psychological Interventions in Cardiac Rehabilitation

Many cardiac rehabilitation programs include psychological interventions such as counseling, which should begin when patients are still in the _____. Increased social support can occur through inclusion of spouses and family in counseling.

III. Coping with Cancer

More than 1 million people a year in the United States are diagnosed with cancer, and many of these people see the diagnosis as a _____ _____ and react with fear, distress, and anxiety.

A. Psychological Impact of Cancer

Cancer patients suffer no more clinical depression than do other hospitalized patients, although distress and acute depression are not uncommon. Nearly all medical treatments for cancer have negative _____ _____ that may add stress to the lives of patients. Surgery, radiation, and _____ all produce unwanted side effects, including changes in body image, loss of hair, nausea, fatigue, weight change, sleep problems, loss of appetite, sex problems, and sterility.

B. Psychological Treatment for Cancer Patients

Psychological interventions have been used to help cancer patients deal with the anger, depression, and anxiety that frequently follow a cancer diagnosis. _____ _____ are especially useful in providing cancer patients with individuals who have faced similar problems and who will offer emotional and informational support. Young cancer patients have special problems in coping with their illness because they often blame _____ for their illness and they may feel responsible for the increased financial hardship of their parents.

IV. Adjusting to Diabetes

Both Type _____ (insulin-dependent) and Type II (noninsulin-dependent) types of diabetes mellitus require changes in lifestyle, including constant monitoring of _____ glucose and strictly complying to the treatment regimen. Type I diabetes requires _____ injections and careful monitoring of _____. Type II, or _____-_____ diabetes does not ordinarily require insulin injections, but it does demand constant and strict compliance to a rigid dietary regimen, regular medical visits, and routine exercise.

A. The Physiology of Diabetes

Diabetes mellitus is a disorder caused by an _____ deficiency. The inability to regulate blood sugar often causes diabetics to develop other health problems such as cardiovascular disease, retina damage, and kidney diseases. If unregulated, diabetes may cause blindness, coma, and even death.

B. The Impact of Diabetes

Although adult-onset diabetes does not usually require insulin injections, it does demand _____ changes as well as oral medication.

C. Health Psychology's Involvement with Diabetes

The diabetics who are particularly poor at complying with the medical and behavioral restrictions are usually _____.

V. Dealing with HIV and AIDS

Acquired immune deficiency syndrome is a disorder produced by the

_____   _____   _____

(HIV), which causes the immune system to lose its effectiveness and leaves the

body defenseless against bacterial, viral, fungal, parasitic, cancerous, and other

_____ diseases.

A. Incidence and Mortality Rates for HIV/AIDS

In 1992, the Centers for Disease Control and Prevention changed the

definition of AIDS, which _____ the number of HIV cases.

Since that time, death rates from AIDS have dramatically

_____ due to AIDS patients _____

_____ and to changes in lifestyle for people at high risk.

B. The HIV and AIDS Epidemics

The four HIV/AIDS epidemics are (1) male-male sexual contact,

(2) _____ _____ use, heterosexual contact, and

(4) transmission from _____ to _____. Of these

four epidemics, the one with the greatest decline in mortality is male-male sexual

contact, while incidence from heterosexual contact is _____ .

C. Symptoms of HIV and AIDS

HIV progresses over a decade or more through _____ stages,

but the first two are not easily identifiable. The third stage involves swollen

lymph nodes, fever, fatigue, night sweats, loss of appetite, loss of weight,

persistent diarrhea, white spots in the mouth, and painful skin rashes. The fourth stage involves a low level of _____ - _____, The two

leading causes of death among AIDS patients are *Pneumocystis carninii*

pneumonia and _____ sarcoma.

D. The Transmission of HIV

The main routes of HIV infection are from person to person through

_____ contact, from mother to child during pregnancy or birth,

and from direct contact with blood or blood products. The largest number of HIV

infections in the United States is still through _____ to

_____ sexual contact, with anal intercourse being especially risky for

the _____ partner. The sharing of unsterilized needles by

_____ drug users allows the direct transmission of infected blood

from one person to another and is the _____ most frequent source

of HIV infection among men in the United States and the most frequent source

for women. The leading source of HIV in Africa, the fastest growing source in the

United States, and the second leading source of HIV infection among women in

the United States is _____ _____. Unsafe

sexual behaviors are situational, and particularly dangerous situations include

those where _____ and other drugs are being used. Other

means of HIV transmission include exposure to infected blood through

transfusions and during the _____ process.

E. Psychologists' Role in the AIDS Epidemic

Psychologists have played several roles in controlling the AIDS epidemic, including counseling with HIV patients, changing _____-_____ behaviors. helping patients cope with deteriorating cognitive abilities, and investigating the behavioral aspects of AIDS. They also attempt to change risky behaviors, such as sharing _____ with an infected person and having _____ sexual contact with an infected person.

VI. Living with Alzheimer's Disease

Alzheimer's disease is a degenerative disease of the _____ and a major source of impairment among older people. Two forms of the disease exist, one that occurs before age 60 and the other after age 70. The more common of the two is the late-onset type, which seems to be related to apolipoprotein E, a _____ involved in cholesterol metabolism. Symptoms of Alzheimer's disease include language problems, memory loss, confusion, wandering, agitation and irritability, sleep disorders, depression, suspiciousness, incontinence, sexual disorders, and loss of ability to perform routine self-care.

A. Helping the Patient

Alzheimer's disease is presently incurable, and drugs have only a limited ability to control this illness. Several psychological interventions are used to enhance patient's _____-_____ memory and help them cope with depression and problems of orientation.

B. Helping the Family

The symptoms of Alzheimer disease are very distressing to family members

who are subjected to emotional outbursts, suspiciousness, anger, and agitation.
As the disease progresses, constant care is required because the Alzheimer's
patient may _____ away from home at all times of the day.
Eventually, they lose their ability to eat, dress, and clean themselves without
help. Psychosocial interventions such as _____ groups often
help caregivers cope with the strain of living with an Alzheimer's patient.

Answers

I.	chronic
I.A.	social support; control
I.B.	identity
II.	exercise; lower
II.A.	smoking; aerobic (regular)
II.B.	depression
II.C.	hospital
III.	death sentence
III.A.	side effects; chemotherapy
III.B.	Support groups; themselves
IV.	I; blood; insulin; diet; noninsulin-dependent
IV.A.	insulin
IV.B.	lifestyle (dietary)
IV.C.	adolescents (teenagers)
V.	human immunodeficiency virus; opportunistic
V.A.	increased; decreased (dropped; declined); living longer
V.B.	injection drug; mother; infant; increasing (rising)
V.C.	four; T-lymphocytes; Kaposi's
V.D.	sexual; male; male; receptive; injection (intravenous); second; heterosexual contact; alcohol; birth
V.E.	high-risk; needles; unprotected
VI.	brain; protein
VI.A.	short-term
VI.B.	wander; support

Multiple Choice Questions

_____ 1. Sylvia, the first case study in this chapter, had many symptoms of Alzheimer's disease, including
   a. elevated blood pressure.
   b. anger.
   c compulsive neatness.
   d. miserliness.

_____ 2. Which of these is NOT a chronic illness?
   a. hypertension
   b. influenza
   c. cancer
   d. Alzheimer's disease

_____ 3. Chronic illnesses persist over a period of time. Most people with a chronic illness
   a. understand this fact.
   b. see their illness as acute.
   c. will eventually be cured of their illness.
   d. both b and c

_____ 4. Compared with people with acute illnesses, those with chronic diseases are less
   a. compliant with medical recommendations.
   b. knowledgeable about treatment.
   c. knowledgeable about their prognosis.
   d. likely to be older.

_____ 5. Eileen has received a diagnosis of breast cancer. Her most effective coping strategy would be to
   a. avoid thinking about her illness.
   b. investigate her family history of breast cancer.
   c. cognitively and emotionally accept her fate.
   d. join a support group.

_____ 6. Charlie, the case study heart patient, experienced a cardiac rehabilitation program similar to most such programs. This included
   a. extended bed rest.
   b. isolation from spouse and children.
   c. a low-fat diet.
   d. tracing his family history for heart disease.

_____ 7. As a health psychologist working in a large hospital's coronary care program, Loraine is MOST likely to
    a. help physicians during surgery.
    b. design and implement exercise programs.
    c. design and implement dietary programs.
    d. help patients adjust to necessary lifestyle changes.

_____ 8. Dean Ornish and his colleges suggest that a diet in which 30% of calories come from fat
    a. may protect against the development of coronary artery damage.
    b. can reverse coronary artery damage without surgery.
    c. both a and b
    d. neither a nor b

_____ 9. Cardiac patients are MOST likely to suffer for the longest time from
    a. depression.
    b. obsessive-compulsive disorder.
    c. paranoia and delusions.
    d. post-traumatic stress disorder.

_____ 10. Avery has experienced a heart attack, which left both him and his wife Lacey fearful about resuming sexual relations. They should know that such fears
    a. are uncommon among heart patients.
    b. are more common among female heart attack patients.
    c. are not justified by research.
    d. are justified, because many heart patients die during sexual relations.

_____ 11. One important difference between medical procedures for cancer and those for heart disease is that cancer treatments
    a. are much more expensive.
    b. result in fewer distressing side effects.
    c. result in more distressing side effects.
    d. are more likely to produce feelings of paranoia.

_____ 12. With regard to survival from cancer,
    a. about 10% of cancer patients survive at least 5 years.
    b. about one third of cancer patients survive at least 5 years.
    c. more than one half of cancer patients survive at least 5 years.
    d. more than two thirds of cancer patients survive at least 10 years.

_____ 13. In general, patients participating in support groups for cancer patients, compared with those receiving standard medical care,
   a. experienced less stress.
   b. had fewer recurrences of cancer.
   c. survived longer.
   d. all of the above

_____ 14. This type of diabetes does NOT usually require insulin injections:
   a. Type I.
   b. Type II.
   c. neither Type I nor Type II.
   d. both Type I and Type II.

_____ 15. Most adults who develop diabetes are
   a. men.
   b. thin.
   c. require insulin injections.
   d. none of the above

_____ 16. This technique shows some promise in helping adolescent diabetics comply with their treatment regimen:
   a. written instructions.
   b. biofeedback.
   c. hypnosis.
   d. threats.

_____ 17. In 1992, the Centers for Disease Control and Prevention changed the definition of HIV infection. This resulted in
   a. an immediate increase in the number of HIV cases.
   b. an immediate decrease in the number of HIV cases.
   c. no change in the number of female HIV cases but an increase in male HIV cases.
   d. no change in the number of female HIV cases but a decrease in male HIV cases.

_____ 18. Since 1994, the death rate from AIDS has
   a. increased sharply.
   b. increased gradually.
   c. remained about the same.
   d. decreased sharply.

_____ 19. During the 1990s, the largest decline in the proportion of HIV cases was
  a. among gay men.
  b. among African American women.
  c. among injection drug users.
  d. among European American women

_____ 20. The recent decline in AIDS mortality is due to a
  a. shorter survival time for AIDS patients.
  b. decline in the incidence of AIDS.
  c. decline in incidence rates of HIV infection for heterosexual women.
  d. an increase in the incidence of HIV infection for heterosexual men.

_____ 21. HIV progresses over a decade or more through four stages, the first of which is characterized by
  a. a CDR+ T-lymphocyte cell count of less than 200.
  b. a period of latency in which the person experiences few, if any symptoms.
  c. symptoms of fever, sore throat, skin rash, and headache.
  d. a cluster of symptoms, including swollen lymph nodes, fever, fatigue, night sweats, and loss of appetite.

_____ 22. The LEAST likely mode of HIV transmission would be
  a. receiving a blood transfusion from someone infected with HIV.
  b. having sexual intercourse with someone who is infected.
  c. sharing eating utensils with someone who is infected.
  d. sharing injection needles with someone who is infected.

_____ 23. Which of these factors is NOT positively associated with unprotected sexual contact among gay men?
  a. heavy use of alcohol
  b. heavy drug use
  c. being 35 years old or older
  d. willingness to engage in other risky behaviors

_____ 24. Recently, the incidence of HIV infection is increasing fastest for
  a. injection drug use among women.
  b. injection drug use among men.
  c. male-female sexual contact.
  d. male-male sexual contact.

_____ 25. The risk for this disease increases sharply with age:
  a. Type I diabetes.
  b. acquired immune deficiency syndrome.
  c. leukemia.
  d. Alzheimer's disease.

_____ 26. Which of these is most likely to be a symptom of Alzheimer's disease?
   a. high blood pressure
   b. wandering and sleep disorders
   c. high cholesterol
   d. enhanced memory for recent events

_____ 27. Vernon, a 68 year old man, has been wandering about his neighborhood at unusual hours of the day. He seems both confused and agitated. For no apparent reason, he strikes out at his wife verbally, though he has never hit her. He has some awareness that his memory is not as good as it once was, and this knowledge frustrates him. These symptoms best describe
   a. AIDS.
   b. Alzheimer's.
   c. attention deficit disorder.
   d. Kaposi's sarcoma.

_____ 28. The chronic illness that is usually the most disruptive to families is
   a. heart disease.
   b. cancer.
   c. AIDS.
   d. Alzheimer's disease.

Multiple Choice Answers

1.	b	15.	d
2.	b	16.	c
3.	b	17.	a
4.	a	18.	d
5.	d	19.	a
6.	c	20.	b
7.	d	21.	c
8.	a	22.	c
9.	a	23.	c
10.	c	24.	c
11.	c	25.	d
12.	c	26.	b
13.	d	27.	b
14.	b	28.	d

Essay Questions

1. What psychological factors are important in the management of diabetes?

2. Evaluate the statement, "With the new drugs developed to treat AIDS, psychologists will play a less important role in the AIDS epidemic."

Good points to include in your essay answers:

1. A. Both types of diabetes mellitus have the psychological impact of living with an incurable disease and require lifestyle changes and self-care in order for these patients to survive and to avoid medical complications.
   1. Living with a chronic disease can produce denial, which can lead diabetics to ignore their condition and to avoid proper self-care.
   2. Diabetics who accept their condition can be angry or resentful, which can also influence their self-care.

   B. Stress is a factor in blood glucose regulation for some diabetics.

   C. Patients' understanding of diabetes and their perception of symptoms affect their behavior, including what symptoms require a response and what response they choose.

   D. The lifestyle changes for diabetes management are a compliance problem that is especially difficult for children and adolescents.
   1. Feeling abnormal or left out of normal activities can be difficult for children and adolescents.
   2. Adhering to a complex regimen of diet, glucose testing, and insulin injections is a difficult regimen to manage.

2. A. The statement is not true because the drugs do not prevent and do not cure HIV infection.
   1. Drugs and medical treatment have made a difference in survival time for those infected with HIV.
   2. The modes of infection are behavioral, and the only way of slowing the spread of infection are behavioral interventions.

   B. Psychologists study behavior, the major mode of transmission of the virus.
   1. Psychologists devise interventions to change high-risk behaviors.
   2. Psychologists study the behavioral manifestations of HIV infection on the central nervous system.

   C. Psychologists also play an important role in providing health care for those with HIV.
   1. Psychologists offer counseling to those who are considering HIV testing to help them cope with the stress of deciding and learning about their HIV status.
   2. Psychologists offer counseling to those who are infected with HIV, helping them manage the distress of the diagnosis.
   3. Psychologists counsel those who are HIV infected so that they will not pass on their infection and so that they will adopt healthier lives.

Let's Get Personal—
How Chronic Illness Changed My Family

To better understand the impact of chronic illness on families, interview someone who has a chronic condition or someone who has lived with a person with a chronic illness. Chronic illness is very common, so finding someone who has lived with chronic illness will not be difficult. You want to determine what impact the illness has had on the individual and on the family.

The following questions will allow you to understand the impact of the condition on the person and on his or her family.

What disorder does the person have?

When was the person initially diagnosed?

What was the person's initial reaction to the diagnosis?

What was required for the person's adjustment to the condition?

How did the family react to the diagnosis?

How has the person's chronic condition changed the way that family members interact with each other?

What other changes have occurred in the family as a result of this person's condition?

What positive changes have occurred as a result of the condition?

What negative changes have occurred as a result of the condition?

How was the experience of living with a chronic illness different than what you imagined before you had the experience?

CHAPTER 12
Preventing Injuries

Fill in the Rest of the Story

I. Unintentional Injuries

Unintentional injuries (accidents) are the fourth leading cause of death in the United States, accounting for about 4% of all deaths. However, among young people 15 to 24, unintentional injuries account for about _____ percent of all deaths. During the past 30 years, death rates from unintentional injuries have _____, but the pattern of death and disability varies by developmental stages.

A. Childhood

Children often suffer unintentional injuries from the unsafe acts of adults. The leading cause of unintentional injuries for children (as well as for people of all ages) is _____ _____ _____. Most motor vehicle-related injuries to children under age 5 are from adult's failure to restrain an infant in the _____ seat of a car. Other frequent causes of unintentional injuries to children include drownings, burns, falls, suffocations, poisonings and _____ mishaps.

B. Youth

Compared with childhood, the ages 15 to 24 are much _____ dangerous. More than 75% of deaths to young adults are due to

_____ _____ _____. Most deaths among
young people are the result of modifiable behaviors, such as riding with a driver
who has been drinking, failure to wear bicycle helmets or motorcycle helmets,
and failure to wear a _____ while riding in an automobile.
The single most important contributor to motor vehicle injuries at all ages is
_____, which both impairs judgment and interferes with
_____ functioning.

C. Adulthood

Death rates from unintentional injuries during adulthood are similar to those
during youth, except that death rates from motor vehicle crashes during ages 25
to 44 are much _____ than for ages 15 to 24. For adults (as well as
youth) _____ is involved in a large number of unintentional
injuries. For older adults, death from motor vehicle crashes account for a smaller
percentage of unintentional deaths, but, like children, older adults have high
rates of unintentional deaths from _____ and fires. In the
workplace, _____ Americans suffer more unintentional injuries
than do _____ Americans, and men have more injuries than
women.

II. Strategies for Reducing Unintentional Injuries

Psychologists have become concerned with unintentional injuries and have
played some role in each of three general strategies for reducing their number,
i. e., changing laws, changing the environment, and changing individual
_____.

A. Changing the Individual's Behavior

Programs to change the individual's behavior have centered around strategies to prevent home injuries, to reduce motor vehicle injuries, and to diminish bicycle injuries. Most programs to prevent home injuries target either elderly people or _____. Most of these programs have had a _____ success rate, as have strategies aimed at preventing workplace injuries through changing behavior. One strategy to reduce motor vehicle injuries through modifying individual behavior is the

_____ _____ program, which has been encouraged by the media, bars, restaurants, and the alcohol industry despite evidence that it increases _____ drinking among adolescents and young adults. Educational programs have had limited effectiveness in increasing use of bicycle _____ among children and young people. Evidence suggests that the availability of low-cost, _____ helmets increases the use of bicycle helmets.

B Changing the Environment

Changing the environment is generally more effective in reducing unintentional injuries than changing _____

_____. Environmental changes include building safer motor vehicles and safer roads as well as making homes and the _____ safer.

C. Changing the Law

Laws mandating safety are generally _____ effective than programs aimed at changing individual behaviors or altering the environment. During the past 50 years, a number of laws were passed in the United States that improved safety. Some of these have included laws requiring _____ - _____ containers such as aspirin bottles, seatbelts and _____ for automobiles, and _____ for bicycle and motorcycle riders.

III. Intentional Injuries

The two leading causes of death from intentional injuries are _____ and homicide. The _____ _____ leads all nations in the rate of intentional injuries.

A. Childhood

Children between ages 5 and 9 have the _____ death rate for any age group, and they are more likely to die from _____ than from intentional injuries. Infants less than a year old have a much _____ rate of homicide than do children 1 to 14. Children of all ages are exposed to violence through the media as well as through witnessing violence in their families and communities.

B. Youth

Suicides rates increase rapidly during adolescence and early adulthood, but _____ is a more common cause of death from intentional injury for

15- to 24-year olds. Both ethnic background and _____ relate to homicide: African Americans are much more likely than European Americans to be murdered, and _____ have higher homicide rates than _____. Thus, the one group that has disproportionate number of homicide victims is young _____ _____

_____.

C. Adulthood

As people in the United States advance through adulthood,

_____ rates drop dramatically, while _____ rates show a gradual increase. A serious problem during adulthood is domestic violence, which is directed mostly against _____. When men dominate their family with acts of violence or threats of violence, a kind of terrorism called _____ terrorism exists.

IV. Strategies to Reduce Intentional Injuries

Strategies to reduce intentional injuries include changing the individual's behavior, changing the environment, and changing the _____. These strategies have been aimed at domestic violence, workplace violence, and community and school violence.

A. Domestic Violence

Strategies to reduce domestic violence have targeted child abuse, partner violence, and abuse of _____ people. Parents at highest risk to abuse their children are often poor, young, and have a history of

_____, either as a victim or perpetrator. Strategies for

preventing partner abuse often include shelters for the abused partner and legal

interventions, which are only partially successful because many abused partners

are reluctant to _____ domestic violence. Strategies for

preventing violence to older people are often similar to those designed to prevent

violence to _____, because people in both groups have

difficulty protecting themselves.

B. Creating Safer Workplaces

Workplaces can be vulnerable to intentional injuries inflicted by spouses who

enter the workplace to harm their spouse (a continuation of domestic violence)

and by workers who act violently against their _____ or

bosses. Companies can create safer workplaces by helping potential victims

escape abusive situations, formulating plans for dealing with dangerous

employees, and sending clear messages that neither verbal _____

nor even trivial levels of violence will be accepted.

C. Reducing Community and School Violence

Violence in communities and schools affect young people as both

_____ and as perpetrators. Many schools have conflict

resolution programs to teach problem-solving skills and violence prevention.

Legal strategies that restrict young people from gaining access to

_____ have some limited success in reducing community and

school violence.

D. Cutting Suicide Rates

Suicide becomes a serious problem as early as 10 years of age and continues

as a problem from adolescence to old age. Some schools have program for

counseling at-risk students and training teachers and students to watch for signs

of _____ ideation in students. Programs for reducing suicide

among older people have had limited success.

Answers

I.	40; declined
I.A.	motor vehicle crashes; back; bicycle
I.B.	more; motor vehicle crashes; seatbelts; alcohol; psychomotor
I.C.	higher; alcohol; falls; African; European
II.	behaviors
II.A.	children; low (limited); designated drive; binge (heavy); helmets; fashionable (attractive)
II.B.	individual behaviors; workplace
II.C.	more; child-proof; airbags; helmets
III.	suicide; United States
III.A.	lowest; unintentional injuries; higher
III.B.	homicide; gender; men; women; African American men
III.C.	homicide; suicide; women; patriarchal
IV.	law
IV.A.	old; abuse (violence); report (prosecute); children
IV.B.	coworkers (fellow workers); threats
IV.C.	victims; weapons (firearms)
IV.D.	suicidal

Multiple Choice Questions

_____ 1. Most college students who frequently drive a motor vehicle while drinking
   a. escalate this practice as they become older—if they become older.
   b. seldom ride with other drivers who have been drinking.
   c. do not allow passengers.
   d. engage in other risky behaviors.

_____ 2. High school students who regularly carry a gun or knife to school
   a. tend to engage in other safe behaviors, such as eating a balance diet.
   b. are less likely than other students to smoke cigarettes.
   c. are more likely than other students to wear seatbelts in motor vehicles without airbags.
   d. often engage in other risky behaviors, such as riding with a driver who has been drinking.

_____ 3. Psychologists prefer the term _unintentional injuries_ rather than _accidents_ because the
   a. causes of accidents cannot be studied scientifically.
   b. term _unintentional injuries_ implies chance or fate.
   c. term _accidents_ implies chance or fate.
   d. the term _unintentional injuries_ limits the event to harm to people and does not include harm to machinery or other objects.

_____ 4. During the past 50 years in the United States, mortality rates
   a. from motor vehicle crashes have increased sharply, while those from other unintentional events have declined.
   b. from both motor vehicle crashes and other unintentional events have increased.
   c. from motor vehicle crashes have decreased, while those from other unintentional events have increased.
   d. from both motor vehicle crashes and other unintentional events have decreased.

_____ 5. Among young people 15 to 24, unintentional injuries, suicides, and violent deaths from homicides are responsible for about what percent of deaths?
   a. 33%
   b. 50%
   c. 75%
   d. 90%

_____ 6. For young people up to age 35, _____ is the leading cause of death in the United States.
   a. homicide
   b. HIV infection
   c. cancer
   d. unintentional injuries

_____ 7. Most fatal and nonfatal injuries in the United States are due to
   a. motor vehicle crashes.
   b. airplane crashes.
   c. weather-related events, such as hurricanes and tornadoes.
   d. fires.

_____ 8. Automobile seatbelts protect drivers from fatal injuries when motorist are driving
   a. large cars.
   b. small cars.
   c. at a slow speed.
   d. at a high speed.
   e. any size car at any speed.

_____ 9. This factor is the single greatest contributor to both fatal and nonfatal unintentional injuries:
   a. careless personalities.
   b. marijuana.
   c. alcohol.
   d. unsafe conditions.

_____ 10. In the United States, people go from a relatively safe age to a very dangerous age when they go from
   a. infancy to childhood.
   b. childhood to adolescence and young adulthood.
   c. adolescence and young adulthood to middle age.
   d. middle age to old age.

_____ 11. High school students engage in many risky behaviors, but fewer students _____ than any other dangerous practice.
   a. wear a helmet while riding a bicycle.
   b. wear a helmet while riding a motorcycle.
   c. use a seatbelt while riding in a car.
   d. ride with a driver who has been drinking.

_____ 12. This factor is most closely related to risky behaviors among high school students:
   a. ethnic background.
   b. level of intelligence.
   c. gender.
   d. geographic location.

_____ 13. Cigarette smokers tend to have more than their share of fire-related injuries and
   a. also more than their share of nonfire-related injuries.
   b. fewer than their share of nonfire-related injuries.
   c. about the same rate of nonfire-related injuries as nonsmokers.
   d. fewer than their share of motor vehicle injuries.

_____ 14. In the United States, death from fire is MOST likely to be related to
   a. arson.
   b. alcohol.
   c. smoking.
   d. lightning.

_____ 15. Which of these strategies is generally the LEAST effective means of reducing fatal and nonfatal unintentional injuries?
   a. enforcement of safety-oriented laws
   b. focus on changing the individual's behaviors
   c. manufacture of safer equipment
   d. emphasis on building a safer environment

_____ 16. Older people, compared with young adults,
   a. have an increased risk of fire-related injuries.
   b. have a decreased risk of suicide.
   c. have an increased risk of homicide.
   d. all of the above

_____ 17 The LEAST effective strategy for reducing unintentional injuries is to
   a. build safer equipment.
   b. change the individual's behavior.
   c. change laws to require safety.
   d. make the environment safer.

_____ 18. Programs to increase children's use of bicycle helmets should
   a. emphasize the dangerous consequences of not wearing a helmet.
   b. emphasize the health consequences of wearing a helmet.
   c. make low-cost, fashionable helmets more available to children.
   d. begin during adolescence when teenagers are old enough to understand the consequence of risky behaviors.

_____ 19. Which of these would be an example of an environmental change designed to reduce unintentional injuries?
   a. having smoke detectors in the home
   b. changing people's beliefs about the usefulness of smoke detectors
   c. passing legislation mandating smoke detectors in every home
   d. all of the above

_____ 20. The first and second leading causes of death in the United States for people 15 to 24 are
   a. suicide and cancer.
   b. cancer and heart disease.
   c. unintentional injuries and homicide.
   d. AIDS and suicide.

_____ 21. The people most likely to be murder victims in the United States are
   a. young African American men.
   b. young African American women.
   c. elderly women.
   d. children below age seven.

_____ 22. With regard to domestic violence, research has found that
   a. nearly 80% of men and 50% of women endorse violence as an acceptable means of solving some problems.
   b. about half the husbands see violence as an acceptable way to solve problems, but only 5% of wives agree with this assessment.
   c. about 30% of the husbands and 25% of the wives studied see violence as an acceptable way to solve some domestic problems.
   d. more women than men regard violence as an acceptable means of solving domestic disputes.

_____ 23. Most sexual assaults in the United States are
   a. committed against African American women.
   b. committed against women ages 25 to 45.
   c. are reported to authorities within the first 24 hours of the attack.
   d. are not reported to authorities.

_____ 24. In the United States, the leading cause of death among people 15 to 24 is unintentional injuries, and the second leading cause is
   a. AIDS.
   b. cancer.
   c. suicide
   d. homicide.

Multiple Choice Answers

1.	d	13.	a
2.	d	14.	c
3.	c	15.	b
4.	d	16.	a
5.	c	17.	b
6.	d	18.	c
7.	a	19.	a
8.	e	20.	c
9.	c	21.	a
10.	b	22.	c
11.	a	23.	d
12.	c	24.	d

Essay Questions

1. Evaluate the strategies for lowering unintentional injuries—altering individual behavior, modifying the environment, or changing the law?

2.   What is the impact of intentional injuries?

Good points to include in your essay answers:

1. A. The strategy of decreasing injury by changing the law has been the most successful of the three.
    1. The exception is legal interventions that punish unsafe behavior, which are usually quite successful provided the penalties for violation of the law are very severe.
    2. The legal interventions that require safety are more successful, including mandates to manufacturers to build safer automobiles and to people to use safety devices such as seatbelts and helmets.
    B. The strategy of decreasing injury by changing the environment has been applied to home and motor vehicle safety, and programs that decrease safety hazards in homes and playgrounds tend to be more effective in reducing minor rather than major hazards.
    C. Programs that attempt to change individual behavior have been the least successful, offering evidence of only marginal success.

2. A. Intentional violence has an impact throughout the lifespan, causing lost years of life and producing developmental problems.
    1. Community violence is a factor for all age groups.
    2. Access to firearms increases the deadliness of violence.
    B. During childhood, homicide is a leading cause of death and intentional violence is a major cause of injury.
    C. For youth, both suicide and homicide are leading causes of death and attempts are a major cause of injury.
    1. The impact is not uniform, and both gender and ethnic background combine to put African American men at heightened risk.
    2. School and community violence are problems that affect youth to a greater extent than others.
    D. For adults, partner abuse and elder abuse are areas of concern

Let's Get Personal—

What Is the Safety Risk?

People often take chances that put their safety at risk, and you are probably no exception. These safety risks involve driving after drinking or riding with a driver who has been drinking, failing to wear seatbelts, and failing to wear motorcycle and bicycle helmets. To better understand the extent of the increased risk involved with these behaviors, research the injury rate and death rate for the following categories:

	Injury Rate	Fatality Rate
An automobile crash involving—		
A drinking driver		
A driver who has not been drinking		
A passenger riding with a drinking driver		
A passenger riding with a driver who has not been drinking		
A driver or passenger who was not wearing a seatbelt		
A driver or passenger who was wearing a seatbelt		
A motorcycle crash involving—		
Someone who is wearing a helmet		
Someone who is not wearing a helmet		
A bicycle crash involving—		
Someone who is wearing a helmet		
Someone who is not wearing a helmet		

CHAPTER 13
Smoking Tobacco

Fill in the Rest of the Story

I. Smoking and the Respiratory System

The respiratory system functions to take oxygen into the body and to

remove _____ _____. Air is taken into the body

through the mouth or nose through contractions of the _____;

from the mouth or nose, it travels past the larynx, down the trachea and

_____ tubes, and into the lungs. Airborne particles such as

smoke and other pollutants easily enter the body through the

_____ system, but the body has several protective

mechanisms, such as sneezing and _____ to expel some of

these dangerous particles. Respiratory disorders of most interest to health

psychologists are the chronic _____ pulmonary diseases of

bronchitis (inflammation of the bronchi) and _____, a chronic

lung disease in which scar tissue and mucus obstruct the respiratory

passages.

The principal drug in tobacco is _____, a stimulant drug

which is extremely toxic in large doses, although its harmful effects on

smokers are hard to measure.

II. A Brief History of Tobacco Use

Although Native Americans smoked tobacco before the voyages of Columbus, when the early European explorers discovered tobacco, they quickly took to the smoking habit. However, cigarettes did not gain popularity until the early years of the _____ century. By 1963, well over _____ the adult males in the United States. were regular cigarette smokers.

III. Choosing to Smoke

People who choose to smoke increase their risk of cardiovascular disease, lung cancer, chronic obstructive pulmonary diseases, and a variety of other diseases.

A. Who Smokes and Who Does Not?

Currently, however, about _____ percent of the adults in the United States smoke, and this percentage has _____ since the 1960s. Although smoking rates for most groups are declining, those of _____ have increased. Currently the best demographic predictor of smoking is _____ level.

B. Why Do People Smoke?

Each year in the United States nearly _____ teenagers begin smoking, and many believe that they can and will quit before they suffer from any of the dangers of smoking. People begin smoking for a variety of reasons, but most begin as _____ when peer pressure is strong. Young people may also see smoking as a means of gaining personal control or of rebelling against adult authority.

People may continue to smoke for several reasons: to increase positive affect, to decrease of _____ feelings, and to satisfy a habit or an addiction. According to the _____ _____ model, people may continue to smoke so they can maintain an adequate level of nicotine and to prevent withdrawal symptoms. Some smokers do develop an addiction to nicotine and will take _____ puffs from low-nicotine cigarettes to acquire the needed amount of _____. The social learning model suggests that people learn to smoke in much the same manner that they learn other social behaviors, namely through positive and negative _____. Reinforcement must outweigh the unpleasant sensations experienced by most first time smokers in order to explain the initiation of smoking.

IV. Health Consequences of Tobacco Use

Cigarette smoking is the leading cause of preventable disease and death in the United States, accounting for about _____ deaths a year and about 20 percent of all deaths.

A. What Is the Evidence?

The relationship between cigarette smoking and declining health is so strong that many scientists are willing to say that a

_____ and _____ relationship exist between

smoking and disease and death. The leading cause of death in the United

States, as well as the primary cause of cigarette-related deaths is

_____ disease. Smoking also plays a role in the development

of several cancers, especially _____ cancer, but it is also

related to cancers of the lip, oral cavity, pharynx, esophagus, pancreas,

larynx, trachea, urinary bladder, and kidney.   Currently, the third

leading cause of death in the United States is _____

_____ _____ disease, and cigarette smoking

accounts for more than _____ percent of these deaths.

B. Other Effects of Smoking

Compared with nonsmokers, smokers tend to have higher rates of

ulcers and diseases of the mouth. They also have _____

wrinkles, _____ physical strength, and are more likely to be ill.

C. Cigar and Pipe Smoking

Cigar and pipe smoking are neither as common nor as

_____ as cigarette smoking, provided that these smokers do

not inhale. Cigars and pipe smokers, however, experience elevated risk of

lung and several other cancers (especially of the mouth, pharynx,

esophagus, and larynx) as well as _____ diseases.

D. Passive Smoking

Exposure to the smoke of other people is called passive smoking or

_____ _____ _____ (ETS). The

relative risk for lung cancer for people exposed to environmental tobacco

smoke is around _____ percent higher than those not

exposed. Compared with this risk for lung cancer, a woman's risk of

developing breast cancer from passive smoking is much

_____. Although the relative risk of passive smoking for

heart disease is about the same as it is for lung cancer, environmental

tobacco smoke claims far _____ victims from heart disease

than from lung cancer. The people at greatest risk from environmental

tobacco smoke are _____.

E. Smokeless Tobacco

Use of smokeless tobacco rose sharply during the 1980s and 1990s

among _____ American teenage boys, who tend to believe

that this form of tobacco is safer than cigarette smoking. However,

smokeless tobacco has been associated with increased rates of

_____ cancer and periodontal disease. Prevention of

smokeless tobacco is usually part of a smoking prevention program and

not a separate intervention.

V. Interventions for Reducing Smoking

Breaking the smoking habit is difficult, because smoking has both a positive and a negative _____ value. Programs aimed at reducing smoking rates can be divided into two types: those that deter people from beginning and those that encourage current smokers to

_____.

A. Deterring Smoking

Adolescents often recognize the dangers of smoking, but they smoke anyway, holding the _____ _____ that they will not be harmed by the habit. The success rates of most educational programs aimed at preventing young people from smoking are

_____. The effects of buffering programs are initially

_____, but they do not persist for years. Multimodal programs that include _____ skills are generally more effective.

B. Quitting Smoking

Although quitting is not easy, about _____ percent of U.S. adults have quit. Most people who have quit smoking have done so

_____ _____ _____. Nicotine replacement therapy provides smokers with progressively lower amounts of nicotine through either nicotine gum or the nicotine _____. Nicotine replacement therapy, which is more effective than a

_____, is often combined with psychological approaches, including behavior _____, cognitive-behavioral techniques, contracts, group therapy, social support, relaxation training, stress management, and "booster" sessions. Smokers who have the support of family members and who believe that they can quit; that is, those with high _____ _____ have higher quit rates than do smokers without these conditions. When certain conditions are NOT considered, _____ have higher quit rates than _____. However, compared to male smokers, female smokers are *less* likely to be married, to have made a previous attempt to quit, to have persisted in quit attempts, and to be heavy smokers and *more* likely to live with a smoker. Each of these conditions presents women with greater obstacles to quitting. In addition to gender, having strong _____ support and a diagnosis of heart disease prompts quitting, whereas heavy use of _____ makes quitting more difficult

C. Relapse Prevention

Many people who quit smoking (or other unhealthy behaviors) equate a single slip with total _____. Nevertheless, relapse need not be permanent, and many smokers continue in cycles of quitting and relapse until they quit permanently.

VI. Effects of Quitting

Quitting smoking is likely to bring about two health-related effects; better health and _____ gain.

A. Quitting and Weight Gain

For most smokers who quit, weight gain is modest, about _____

pounds. For others, however, weight gain may be quite large, but not

large enough to cancel the health benefits of quitting.

B. Health Benefits of Quitting

By quitting smoking, both men and women can increase their

_____ expectancy, quickly decrease their risk of

_____ disease, and more slowly decrease their risk for

_____ cancer.

Answers

I.   carbon dioxide; diaphragm; bronchial; respiratory; coughing;
        obstructive; emphysema; nicotine
II.   20th; half (50%)
III.A. 25; declined (decreased); adolescents (teenagers); educational
III.B   700,000; teenagers (adolescents); negative; nicotine addiction;
        more; nicotine; reinforcement
IV.   400,000
IV.A.   cause; effect; cardiovascular (heart); lung; chronic obstructive
        pulmonary; 80
IV.B.   more; less
IV.C.   dangerous (harmful); cardiovascular
IV.D.   environmental tobacco smoke; 30; higher; more; children (infants)
IV.E.   European; oral
V.   reinforcement; quit (stop)
V.A.   optimistic bias; low; strong; refusal
V.B.   25; on their own (without professional help); patch; placebo;
        modification; self-efficacy; men; women; social; alcohol
VI.C.   relapse
VI.   weight
VI.A.   10
VI.B.   life; heart; lung

Multiple Choice Questions

_____ 1. Through the respiratory system, the body takes in oxygen and eliminates
a. nitrogen.
b. methane.
c. carbon dioxide.
d. nitrogen and carbon dioxide.

_____ 2. Anna coughs whenever she first inhales cigarette smoke. Anna should know that coughing
a. is a probable sign of lung cancer.
b. is nature's way of expelling irritants from the respiratory tract.
c. draws oxygen more deeply into the lungs.
d. is a certain symptom of bronchitis.

_____ 3. The percentage of adults in the United States who smoke is currently declining from the peak it reached
a. during the Civil War.
b. during the 1920s.
c. during the 1960s.
d. during the 1980s.

_____ 4. The current decline in smoking rates can be traced to
a. the effectiveness of hypnosis in smoking cessation programs.
b. the 1964 Surgeon General's report.
c. the 1985 ban on depicting smoking in Hollywood movies.
d. the failure of tobacco companies to achieve their goal of appearing as good corporate citizens.

_____ 5. Since 1970, cigarette smoking has declined most sharply for
a. adult men.
b. adult women.
c. adolescent boys.
d. adolescent girls.

_____ 6. During the 1990s, smoking rates for adolescents showed
a. an increase for both girls and boys.
b. a decrease for both girls and boys.
c. an increase for girls and a decrease for boys.
d. an increase for boys and a decrease for girls.

_____ 7. Which factor has the strongest inverse relationship to smoking rates?
a. age
b. weight
c. level of psychological well-being
d. educational level

_____ 8. Blanca smokes about 30 cigarettes a day. When she is NOT smoking, she is very much aware of this fact. According to Tomkin's model, Blanca is probably
a. an addictive smoker.
b. a negative affect smoker.
c. a positive affect smoker.
d. a habitual smoker.

_____ 9. What is the best answer to the question of why people smoke?
a. People smoke so they have something to do with their hands.
b. People smoke because it is a habit they cannot break.
c. People smoke in order to lose weight.
d. People smoke for a variety of reasons.

_____ 10. Palmer is 15 years old and has been smoking for 2 years. Although he is familiar with most of the known risks of cigarette smoking, Palmer believes that these hazards apply to other people and not to him. Palmer is exhibiting
a. an extraverted personality.
b. an introverted personality.
c. an optimistic bias.
d. a pessimistic bias.

_____ 11. Nicotine
a. is a tranquilizer.
b. can be addictive.
c. is relatively harmless even in large quantities.
d. all of the above

_____ 12. Sales of American tobacco companies are likely to remain strong
a. because tobacco markets in African, Eastern Europe, and Asia are expanding.
b. because tobacco companies are now using subliminal advertising to motivate young people to begin smoking.
c. because former cigarette smokers are switching to cigars and pipes, which consume more tobacco than do cigarettes.
d. more middle age and older adults are beginning to smoke.

_____ 13. Evidence that cigarette smoking is a greater risk than environmental pollution for lung cancer comes from studies that found
a. an increase in lung cancer among nonsmokers.
b. a relatively stable pattern of lung cancer among nonsmokers and an increase of lung cancer among smokers.
c. a decrease in lung cancer among male smokers.
d. a decrease in lung cancer among female smokers.

_____ 14. Smokers are most likely to die of lung cancer, heart disease, and chronic obstructive pulmonary disease (COPD). Although more smokers die from _____, the relative risk for _____ is higher, and more than 80 percent of deaths from _____ result from smoking.
a. lung cancer. . . heart disease. . . COPD
b. COPD. . . heart disease. . . lung cancer
c lung cancer. . . COPD. . . heart disease
d. COPD. . . lung cancer. . . heart disease
e. heart disease. . . lung cancer. . . COPD

_____ 15. Which of these conditions is positively related to cigarette smoking?
a. sexual potency among men
b. increased facial wrinkling for men and women
c. recurrence of ulcers
d. all of the above
e. only b and c

_____ 16. Compared with cigarette smokers, people who smoke only a pipe
a. have less than one third the risk of dying from lung cancer.
b. have about the same risk of dying from lung cancer.
c. have less than 2% the risk of dying from lung cancer.
d. have a slightly increased risk of dying from lung cancer.

_____ 17. Research suggests that passive smoking is responsible for
a. more deaths from lung cancer than from heart disease.
b. more deaths from heart disease than from lung cancer.
c. an equal number of deaths from each disease.
d. no deaths from either disease.

_____ 18. Although people in this group do not have an increased risk of lung cancer mortality from passive smoking, they suffer the most adverse overall health affects from environmental tobacco smoke:
a. infant children of smoking parents.
b. wives of smoking husbands.
c. husbands of smoking wives.
d. older parents of smoking children.

_____ 19. Which of these tactics is generally most effective in deterring young people from smoking?
a. warnings on cigarette packs
b. educational procedures
c. threats of illness and early death
d. inoculation programs

_____ 20. You and your classmates begin a comprehensive researched-based smoking inoculation program in the local junior high school. Half of the young students receive the inoculation treatment and half receive only educational pamphlets. At the end of 4 years, you would expect
a. smoking rates in both groups to increase on a year-to-year basis.
b. smoking rates in the treatment group to be lower than rates in the control group.
c. smoking rates in the treatment group to decline while those in the control group rise.
d. both a and b
e. both b and c

_____ 21. Compared with quit rates from a placebo patch, the quit rates from a nicotine patch are
a. about 10% lower.
b. about the same.
c. more than twice as high.
d. more than 10 times higher.

_____ 22. Most smokers who have successfully quit
a. did so through hypnosis.
b. did so on their own.
c. used the nicotine patch.
d. used the nicotine inhaler.

_____ 23. On average, if a man with no heart disease were to follow a diet of no more than 10% of calories from saturated fat, he would extend his life a matter of a few weeks. If the same man were to quit smoking, he would extend his life by
a. about the same length of time.
b. about 3 or 4 months.
c. about 3 or 4 years.
d. about 10 to 20 years.

_____ 24. Henrietta has been a light smoker for about 20 years. If she quits smoking, her mortality risk will
a. be unaffected.
b. return to that of a nonsmoker in about 2 to 3 years.
c. return to that of a nonsmoker in about 16 years.
d. increase due to a change in lifestyle.

Multiple Choice Answers

1.	c	13.	b
2.	b	14.	e
3.	c	15.	e
4.	b	16.	a
5.	a	17.	b
6.	a	18.	a
7.	d	19.	d
8.	a	20.	d
9.	d	21.	c
10.	c	22.	b
11.	b	23.	c
12.	a	24.	c

Essay Questions

1. Is passive smoking as dangerous as smoking?

2. Are the nicotine replacement therapies more successful than other methods of quitting smoking?

Good points to include in your essay answers:

1. A. Passive smoking or environmental tobacco smoke (ETS) is not an equal
    risk for all, and children are at more danger from passive smoking than are
    adults.
       1.   Infants who live with smokers are at increased risk of respiratory
       diseases.
       2.   Smoking is a danger for the unborn, being associated with low birth
       weight.
       3.   The dangers decrease after children pass age 2 years.
    B. For adults, ETS is irritating and annoying but poses only minor health
    risks.
       1.   The risk of lung cancer is slightly elevated by passive smoking.
       2.   The risk of heart disease is elevated by ETS, which presents a more
       pervasive risk than that from lung cancer.

2. A. Nicotine replacement therapy has become a popular treatment for
    smoking.
       1.   Nicotine replacement therapy has two forms: nicotine chewing gum
       and nicotine patches.
       2.   Nicotine replacement is sometimes used as the sole treatment and is
       sometimes combined with other treatment components in a multimodal
       program.
       3.   Nicotine chewing gum is not very effective by itself, but it is more
       effective than a placebo and can be quite effective when combined with
       behavioral therapy.
       4.   Nicotine patches are more popular than the chewing gum and are
       also more effective. They are more than twice as effective as patch
       placebos.
    B. Multimodal behavioral therapy is more effective than nicotine
    replacement therapy alone.
    C. The most effective approach to quitting smoking remains quitting
    without therapy.

Let's Get Personal—

Risk from Smoke Exposure

Most college students do not smoke, thus avoiding the risks associated with cigarettes. A more common smoking-related risk is exposure to passive smoke, and many people are exposed under a variety of circumstances. Evaluate the degree of risk for exposure to various types of smoke, and examine your smoking habits and exposure in the various categories. Compared with nonsmokers, what is the risk of

Lung cancer for smokers?

Lung cancer for nonsmoking spouses of smokers?

Lung cancer for nonsmokers who work with smokers?

Heart disease for smokers?

Heart disease for nonsmoking spouses of smokers?

CHAPTER 14
Using Alcohol and Other Drugs

Fill in the Rest of the Story

I. Alcohol Consumption—Yesterday and Today

The use of alcohol is as old as civilization, and the consumption of alcohol has brought both problems and benefits.

A. A Brief History of Alcohol Consumption

In colonial America drinking was much more common than it is today, partially because _____ and milk were not always purified. The Puritans objected to _____ but not drinking. Alcohol consumption in the United States _____ sharply after 1830 and rose after the _____ _____ was repealed in 1934 by the 21st Amendment.

B. The Prevalence of Alcohol Consumption Today

About _____ percent of the adults in the United States are classified as current drinkers (defined as having at least one drink during the past 30 days), about 15 percent engage in _____ drinking (five or more drinks on the same occasion at least once during the past 30 days), and a little more than 5 percent are _____ drinkers (five or more drinks on the same occasion on at least five different days during the past month) Younger people

223

drink more than older people, and they are more likely to _____ drink. Of the various ethnic groups in the United States, Asian American and _____ Americans have the highest rates of alcohol consumption, and Hispanic Americans and _____ Americans the lowest rates. Educational level is _____ related to amount of alcohol consumption.

II. The Effects of Alcohol

The specific alcohol used in beverages, which is a poison and can cause sudden death when consumed in large quantities, is called _____. Alcohol is one of the drugs that can lead to a situation in which progressively more of the drug is required to produce a constant effect. In other words, alcohol can produce _____. It can also produce dependence and _____ symptoms in the form of delirium tremens. The combination of dependence and withdrawal symptoms is referred to as _____.

A. Hazards of Alcohol

Alcohol does produce a variety of hazards, both direct and indirect. One direct hazard is the accumulation of fat in the liver, which may eventually lead to _____, a major cause of deaths among alcoholics. Prolonged, heavy drinking can also cause neurological damage, and _____ syndrome, which results in severe memory loss and cognitive dysfunction. Heavy drinkers may have a slight increase in risks for cancer of the esophagus, stomach, and liver, Women who drink two to five drinks a day have about a 40%

increased risk for _____ cancer. In large doses, alcohol can

impair the heart's ability to function properly, lead to hypertension, and cause

stroke. Women who drink excessively during pregnancy sometimes give birth to

an infant with _____ _____ syndrome, a disorder

that includes growth deficiencies, central nervous system dysfunction, and

mental retardation. All those harmful consequences that result from alcohol's

effects on coordination and from effects on the processes of aggression,

judgment, and attention are called _____ hazards. The

largest number of alcohol-related deaths is from _____

_____ crashes. In addition, alcohol is involved in about two-thirds

of the homicides in the United States.

B. Benefits of Alcohol

Several studies have reported a J-shaped relationship between alcohol

consumption and health, with nondrinkers and heavy drinkers at an

_____ risk. Most of the benefits of light to moderate drinking

come from reduced _____ disease, which offsets increased risk

from other sources of mortality. The decrease in CHD mortality seems to be due

to increases in _____ - _____ lipoprotein.

III. Why Do People Drink?

Several models have been suggested to explain why people drink.

Historically, the _____ model has had the greatest influence on

therapies for alcohol addiction.

A. The Disease Model

During the past 50 years, the medical profession has advocated a

_____ model of alcoholism. One model, which is more

flexible than the traditional disease model, emphasizes impaired control instead

of loss of control or the inability to abstain. According to this model—called the

_____ _____ model, seven

components make up a syndrome of drinking-related behaviors: (1) narrowing

of drinking repertoire, (2) salience of _____-seeking behavior, (3)

increased _____, (4) withdrawal symptoms, (5) avoidance of

withdrawal by more _____ (6) subjective awareness of the need

to drink, and (7) reinstatement of _____ after abstinence.

Disease models offer a reasonable explanation for why some people drink too

much, but they are less successful in giving reasons why people _____

to drink. Some research suggests that craving for alcohol results from drinkers'

_____ of alcohol's effects, rather than from physical

properties of alcohol.

B. Cognitive-Physiological Theories

Several alternatives to the disease model emphasize the combination of

physiological and _____ changes that occur with alcohol use. The

tension reduction hypothesis assumes that people drink as a means of coping

with _____. Alcohol is a _____ drug, so it is

capable of producing physiological relaxation and slowed reactions. However,

alcohol stimulates some responses, such as _____

_____ and others, such as pulse wave velocity, are

_____. A reformulation of the tension reduction hypothesis,

called the stress-response-dampening effect, showed that alcohol

_____ the strength of responses to stress. When people

drink, thoughts become more _____, which allows people to

reduce or avoid self-statements that would otherwise increase tension. The

notion that alcohol creates effects on social behaviors that produce a kind of

shortsightedness while blocking out insightful cognitive processing is called

_____ _____.

C. The Social Learning Model

Many psychologists have accepted social learning theory, which suggests

that drinking behavior is _____; that is, it is acquired

through positive or negative _____, cognitive mediation, and

by observing others; that is through _____. Social learning

theory assumes that people can also learn to abstain or to drink in moderation.

Thus the goal of treatment might be either abstinence or _____

drinking.

IV. Changing Problem Drinking

Gender is a strong predictor of who will seek treatment for alcoholism,

with _____ far out-numbering _____.

A. Change without Therapy

Many people quit drinking without going into a treatment program. The

term _____ _____ applies to disease cure with

without treatment, but for those who do not consider problem drinking a

disease, this term is not adequate. The term _____ change may

be more accurate, but this too may be misleading because most problems

drinkers who quit without formal treatment have had the help of family and

friends. For people who stop on their own, about _____ percent are

successful.

B. Treatments Oriented toward Abstinence

All treatment programs have _____ as their immediate

goal, although some include controlled drinking as an ultimate goal. Probably

the most common treatment approach in the United States, and one that is

often included as an adjunct to other abstinence programs is

_____ _____, but this program produces a

higher _____ rate than other treatment programs, as well as

more participants likely to binge drink. AA works better for men of

_____ educational levels with strong needs for authoritarianism,

dependence, and sociability. Some alcohol treatment programs include

_____ (Antabuse) or other drugs that interact with alcohol to

produce unpleasant effects. The major problem with this type of therapy is

_____: Patients are not eager to take a drug that will make

them sick if they drink alcohol. A type of therapy based on the classical

conditioning model that combines an electric shock and some other aversive

stimulus to countercondition the patient's response to alcohol is called

_____ _____. Such programs have high

_____ rates and are only marginally effective.

C. Controlled Drinking

During the past 30 years, therapists have observed that a small percentage

of recovered alcoholics were able drink in a _____ fashion, even

in programs aimed at _____. Research shows that programs

teaching control are generally _____ effective than those aimed

at abstinence. In addition, many former problems drinkers have learned on

their own to control consumption. Nevertheless, controlled drinking remains a

controversial issue and is rarely a treatment goal in the _____

_____, but controlled drinking is a more common goal in the United

Kingdom and Australia. Controlled drinking is not an acceptable goal for all

problem drinkers, especially for _____ people with a long history

of problem drinking.

D The Problem of Relapse

Relapse rates for alcohol treatment are almost identical to those for drug

abuse or _____. Most relapse training programs are aimed at changing _____ so that the addict comes to believe that one slip

does *not* equal total relapse.

V. Other Drugs

In the United States illicit drugs have created more

_____ problems than health problems.

A. Health Effects

Potential health hazards are not limited to illicit drugs;

_____ drugs can also pose a risk. Included in the list of legal

drugs are _____ that induce relaxation by lowering the

activity of the brain and even slowing metabolic rate. Sedative drugs include

tranquilizers and alcohol, which have additive effects that make them

dangerous when taken in combination or in large amounts. Barbiturates are

synthetic drugs used medically to induce _____, but used

recreationally to induce euphoria or intoxication. Morphine, heroin, and other

_____ drugs have been used medically to relieve pain, but

they produce both tolerance and dependence after only a short time. Drugs that

produce alertness, reduce feelings of fatigue, elevate mood, decrease appetite,

and include amphetamines are classified as _____ drugs.

Cocaine acts as a stimulant to the _____ system, and the

strength and duration of its action depend on both dose and mode of

administration. The most commonly used illegal drug in the United States is

_____, which has also been used medically to prevent the

vomiting associated with chemotherapy and to treat the eye disease called

_____. Some people use anabolic steroids to increase

_____ bulk or to improve appearance, but medically, steroids

are used to reduce inflammation and to control some allergic reactions.

B. Drug Misuse and Abuse

All psychoactive drugs, including those used primarily for

_____ purposes, are potentially dangerous. When people take

drugs in an inappropriate but not health-threatening manner, they

_____ that drug; they _____ a drug when their

consumption is frequent, heavy, and harmful to their health.

C. Treatment for Drug Abuse

Treatment for illegal drug abuse is similar to the treatment for

_____ abuse. The immediate goal for both is

_____, but the detoxification phase of inpatient treatment is

usually shorter for drug abusers. As with alcohol treatments, programs for drug

abuse suffer from high _____ rates.

D. Preventing and Controlling Drug Use

Drug prevention programs that rely on scare tactics, moral training, factual

information about drug risks, and boosting self-esteem generally have

_____ success rates, but peer-led programs that teach avoidance

of social situations involving drugs are more successful.

Answers

I.A.   water; drunkenness; dropped; 18th Amendment
I.B.   50; binge; heavy; binge; European; African; positively
II.   ethanol; tolerance; withdrawal; addiction
II.A. cirrhosis; Korsakoff; breast; fetal alcohol; indirect; motor vehicle
II.B. increased (elevated); cardiovascular (heart); high-density
III.   disease
III.A. medical; alcohol dependency; drink; tolerance; drinking; dependence; begin; expectation
III.B. cognitive; tension (stress); sedative (depressant); heart rate; slowed (decreased); decreases; superficial; alcohol myopia
III.C. learned; reinforcement; modeling; controlled
IV.   men; women
IV.A. spontaneous remission; unassisted; 20
IV.B. abstinence; Alcoholics Anonymous; dropout; lower; disulfiram; compliance; aversion therapy; dropout
IV.C. controlled; abstinence; more; United States; older
IV.D. smoking; cognitions (beliefs or perceptions)
V.   social
V.A.   legal; sedatives; sleep; opiate; stimulant; nervous; marijuana; glaucoma; muscle
V.B.   medical; misuse; abuse
V.C.   alcohol; abstinence; relapse (dropout)
V.D.   low (limited)

Multiple Choice Questions

_____ 1. A man who drinks one to three drinks a day is considered a
   a. light drinker.
   b. light to moderate drinker.
   c. heavy drinker.
   d. binge drinker.

_____ 2, In the United States, the peak consumption of alcohol occurred
   a. around 1820.
   b. during the Civil War.
   c. during Prohibition.
   d. during the 1960s
   e. during the early 1990s.

_____ 3. In the United States
   a. about 90% of the people drink alcohol, about 40% are binge drinkers, and about 20 are heavy drinkers.
   b. about 75% of the people drink alcohol, and about half of these abuse alcohol.
   c. about half the population are drinkers, 15% are binge drinkers, and 5% are heavy drinkers.
   d. about one-third of the population abuse alcohol to the point that it interferes with their health.

_____ 4. Which group has the highest rate of alcohol consumption in the Unites States?
   a. young and middle-aged adults
   b. women
   c. older adults
   d. young adolescents

_____ 5. Seymour finds himself drinking more in order to maintain the same effects of alcohol. The term that best describes Seymour's condition is
   a. tolerance.
   b. withdrawal.
   c. physical dependence.
   d. psychological dependence.

_____ 6. Celeste has a long history of heavy drinking. She finds herself needing to have a drink in order to go to work, to talk to her sister, to sleep, or to do about anything else. The term that best describes Celeste's condition is
   a. tolerance.
   b. dependence.
   c. withdrawal.
   d. psychological tolerance.

_____ 7. Benita has recently quit drinking after years of alcohol abuse. Now she finds herself restless, irritable, agitated, and shaky. Benita is experiencing
   a. tolerance.
   b. psychological dependence.
   c. physiological dependence.
   d. withdrawal symptoms.

_____ 8. Drugs that produce dependence and that, when discontinued, result in withdrawal symptoms are called
   a. addictive drugs.
   b. psychoactive drugs.
   c. tolerance drugs
   d. illicit drugs.

_____ 9. Claude has a long history of excessive and chronic alcohol abuse and now has confusion, poor memory for recent events, and severe disorientation. Claude is exhibiting symptoms of
   a. aldehyde dehydrogenase psychosis.
   b. psychological withdrawal.
   c. delirium tremens.
   d. Korsakoff syndrome.

_____ 10. Heavy consumption of alcohol generally
   a. decreases a woman's fertility.
   b. increases a woman's fertility.
   c. has no effect on a woman's fertility.
   d. leads to higher birth weight of the baby.
   e. both b and d

_____ 11. Which of the following is an indirect effect of alcohol?
   a. increased high-density lipoprotein cholesterol
   b. increased risk of cirrhosis of the liver
   c. increased risk of unintentional injuries
   d. increased risk of heart disease

_____ 12. Research on the relationship between alcohol consumption and death rate shows
   a. a J-shaped or U-shaped relationship.
   b. a W-shaped relationship.
   c. a direct and dose-response relationship between level of drinking and chances of mortality.
   d. an inverse relationship between level of drinking and chances of mortality.

_____ 13. The type of alcohol that confers some protection against heart disease is
   a. red wine.
   b. white wine.
   c. beer.
   d. liquor.
   e. all alcohol; ethanol itself seems to be the protective ingredient.

_____ 14. Research shows that alcohol may confer some protection against heart disease because it
   a. lowers low-density lipoprotein.
   b. raises low-density lipoprotein.
   c. lowers high-density lipoprotein.
   d. raises high-density lipoprotein.

E #4

_____ 15. The disease model of alcohol consumption has been
   a. embraced by most psychologists for the past 50 years.
   b. embraced by the U.S. medical community for the past 50 years.
   c. abandoned by the majority of those who provide treatment for problem drinking.
   d. both a and b

_____ 16. Using the balanced placebo design, Marlatt and his colleagues found
   a. that alcoholics can be divided into three distinct groups.
   b. support for the tension reduction hypothesis.
   c. that intoxication can be more dangerous than had been previously observed.
   d. that the intoxication experienced from light to moderate drinking is strongly affected by expectancy.

_____ 17. Which of these concepts is NOT part of the alcohol dependency syndrome?
   a. loss of control
   b. narrowing of drinking repertoire
   c. salience of drinking behavior
   d. subjective awareness of the compulsion to drink
   e. all of the above

E 4

_____ 18. For many people, consumption of alcohol impairs their view of reality and changes the way they think about self, stress, and social anxiety. This describes
   a. the stress-response-dampening effect.
   b. gamma alcoholism.
   c. delta alcoholism.
   d. alcohol myopia.

_____ 19. The social learning model of drinking includes these terms:
   a. loss of control, inability to abstain, and disease.
   b. coping, modeling, and negative reinforcement.
   c. stress-response-dampening effect and delta alcoholic.
   d. increased tissue tolerance and adaptive cell metabolism.

_____ 20. People who drink in order to avoid the aversive consequences of abstinence are demonstrating

E #4

    a. alcohol myopia.
    b. positive reinforcement.
    c. negative reinforcement.
    d. the balanced placebo effect.

_____ 21. Another term for quitting drinking without the aid of therapy is
    a. assisted change.
    b. stress-response dampening effect.
    c. spontaneous remission.
    d. disulfiram.

_____ 22. Alcohol abusers who are MOST likely to return to controlled drinking are
    a. young, married people who believe that controlled drinking is a possible goal for them.
    b. older, married people who have at least a 40-year history of heavy drinking.
    c. people who have adopted the philosophy of Alcoholics Anonymous.
    d. people who have tried a variety of treatment approaches and who believe that they are physically dependent on alcohol.

_____ 23. One year after the end of treatment, about 35% of people completing a treatment program for _____ will still be abstinent.
    a. alcohol abuse
    b. opiate abuse
    c. smoking
    d. any of the above

_____ 24. Drugs that change the brain's chemistry, have side effects, and change perception
    a. are all regulated by the FDA.
    b. are specifically excluded from FDA regulation.
    c. are called sedatives.
    d. have crossed the blood-brain barrier.

_____ 25. Which of these drugs can produce both tolerance and dependence in as little as one day?
    a. opiates
    b. anabolic steroids
    c. benzodiazepines
    d. all of the above

_____   26. The combination of cocaine and alcohol
   a.   cancel the effects of each other, posing less danger than either taken separately.
   b.   produces cocaethylene, a potentially deadly chemical, making the combination more dangerous than either separately.
   c.   accounts for approximately 50% of the cases of people admitted to hospital emergency rooms.
   d.   both b and c

Multiple Choice Answers

1.	b	14	d
2.	a	15.	b
3.	c	16.	d
4.	a	17.	a
5.	a	18.	d
6.	b	19.	b
7.	d	20.	c
8.	a	21.	c
9.	d	22.	a
10.	a	23.	d
11.	c	24.	d
12.	a	25.	a
13.	e	26.	b

Match these researchers to their research:

1. Jay Hull

   a. researched the balanced placebo design to assess expectancy effects and alcohol.

2. G. Alan Marlatt and his colleagues

   b. found that some alcoholics were able to resume normal drinking.

3. Claude Steele and his colleagues

   c. developed the self-awareness model to explain drinking.

4. E. M. Jellinek

   d. researched the hereditary basis of alcohol abuse.

5. Donald Goodwin and his colleagues

   e. was a proponent of the disease model of alcoholism.

6. Stanton Peele

   f. conducted a famous and controversial study on controlled drinking.

7. D. L. Davies

   g. contended that researchers have ignored alcohol's benefits.

8. Linda Sobel and Mark Sobel

   h. developed the concept of alcohol myopia.

1. c   2. a   3. h   4. e   5. d   6. g   7. b   8. f

The Balanced Placebo and Alcohol Expectancy Effects

   The balanced placebo design has been important in separating expectancy effects from the pharmacological effects of alcohol. Demonstrate your understanding of this design by filling in the missing information from this figure of the balanced placebo design.

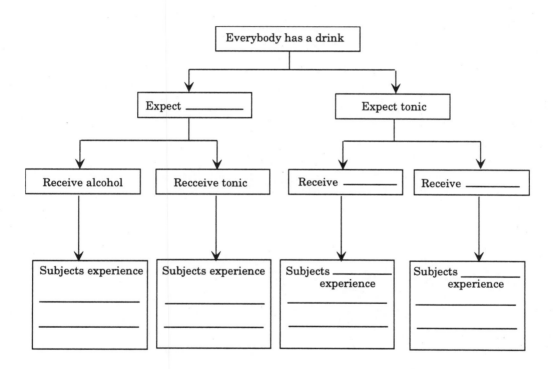

Essay Questions

1. Evaluate the statement, "There is both good news and bad news for people who drink."

2. Two 18-year-old high school seniors grew up in the same neighborhood. One young woman drinks and the other does not. Using the social learning model, explain the difference.

Good points to include in your essay answers:

1. A. The benefits outweigh the hazards for some patterns of drinking, whereas the hazards are more prominent for other patterns of drinking.
    B. Heavy drinking is more of a risk than a benefit.
        1. People who drink heavily on a daily basis are more likely to experience the direct effects of alcohol—liver damage, Korsakoff's syndrome, and fetal alcohol syndrome.
        2. Those who binge drink are at risk from the indirect effects of alcohol, including a variety of unintentional injuries, suicide, and homicide.
    C. Light and moderate drinking can bring greater benefits than risks.
        1. The risks of drinking still apply to these people, but the benefits can outweigh the risks.
        2. The main benefits come from lowered cardiovascular mortality.
        3. Light and moderate drinkers also experience lowered rates of physical illness and hospitalization as well as better mental health.

2   A. The social learning model conceptualizes drinking as learned behavior, similar to other learned behaviors.
        1. People who drink must find reinforcement in drinking or some stimuli associated with it or they would not drink.
        2. People who do not drink find more aversive than positive consequences in drinking, leading them to avoid drinking.
    B. For the young woman who drinks, the social learning model explains her drinking in terms of a greater balance of positive than aversive consequences. Many possibilities exist or combine to make her a drinker.
        1. She may have friends who encourage her drinking.
        2. She may enjoy going to places where drinking is the expected norm.
        3. She may like the taste of alcohol or the feeling of being intoxicated.
        4. She may be trying to cultivate an image that is consistent with drinking.
    C. For the young woman who does not drink, the social learning model explains that behavior in terms of a greater balance of negative than positive consequences associated with drinking.
        1. She may have negative physical reactions to alcohol, similar to the reaction that some Asians experience.
        2. She may not like the taste of alcohol.
        3. She may not like the feeling of intoxication.
        4. She may believe that drinking is wrong for moral or religious reasons.
        5. She may have friends or family whom she wishes to please who disapprove of drinking.

Let's Get Personal—
How Do You Drink?

Drinking alcohol is a common practice for college students, and some college activities are oriented around drinking. College students, however, make a variety of choices concerning their intake of alcohol, with some choosing to abstain, some choosing light or moderate drinking, and others choosing binge or heavy drinking. What are your drinking habits? Examine your drinking pattern by answering these questions:

Do you drink alcohol?

Under what circumstances do you drink—at parties, when you go out, with meals at restaurants, with meals at home, after school or work, or some combination of these circumstances?

On how many days during the past month did you have anything to drink?

Was there one or more occasion during the past year on which you had five or more drinks?

When was the last time that you were intoxicated?

Regardless of your choices, your drinking habits have health implications. If you do not drink, you do not experience the risks associated with increased chances for unintentional injuries, but neither do you experience the potential cardiovascular and other health benefits. If you are a light or moderate drinker, you may receive benefits from your drinking patterns, but you also experience risks resulting from increased chances for unintentional injuries. The benefits may outweigh the risks, but drinking always carries some risk. If you drink heavily or in binges, you probably raise your risks for unintentional injury and liver damage more than you lower your cardiovascular and other health risks.

If your drinking does not conform to the pattern that confers benefits, what would you need to do to drink at that level? Is this a change you want to make?

CHAPTER 15
Eating to Control Weight

Fill in the Rest of the Story

I. The Digestive System

The digestive system begins in the _____, where food is ground into small particles and mixed with saliva from the salivary glands. After swallowing, food is propelled through the esophagus and into the stomach by a process called _____ . Absorption of nutrients does not occur until food reaches the _____ _____. Bile salts produced in the _____ and stored in the gall bladder break down fat molecules. Vitamins are manufactured and absorbed in the _____ _____, and there the fluid volume of the mixture is decreased. Hunger and eating have brain components in the hypothalamus where the lateral hypothalamus. Damage to the lateral hypothalmus _____ eating whereas damage to the ventromedial hypothalamus is related to feelings of _____.

II. Factors in Weight Maintenance

The weight equation consists of three factors: calories eaten, calories used in basal metabolism, and calories expended through _____

_____.

A. Experimental Starvation

A study by Ancel Keys and his associates on experimental starvation indicated that the body slows _____ to adjust for caloric

restriction. Many of the volunteers in Key's study had difficulty

_____ weight, and they experienced irritability, increased

aggression, increased apathy as well as loss of sexual interest and lethargy as a

result of the food restriction. When these men were permitted to eat as much as

they wanted, most regained their lost weight and many remained

_____ with food and regained more weight than they had lost.

B. Experimental Overeating

A study by Ethan Allen Sims and his associates on overfeeding reported that

prison volunteers found overeating _____ and weight gain

increasingly _____.

III. Overeating and Obesity

Because individual differences in metabolism allow some people burn

_____ faster than others, overeating and _____ are not

perfectly related.

A. What Is Obesity?

Determining obesity is not easy, either by definition or by measurement

techniques. A comparison of weight to the charts of the Metropolitan Life

Insurance Company omits any measurement of percent of _____

_____. The skinfold and water immersion techniques are more accurate

in determining fat but are more awkward to use. The _____

_____ index has been used more recently by researchers to determine distribution of weight. Standards for obesity have changed throughout history. Currently in the United States, thinness is valued, but _____ has increased by one-third during the past 20 years.

B. Why Are Some People Obese?

Several models have attempted to explain obesity, including the _____ model, which holds that weight is regulated by a type of internal thermostat that makes fluctuations in either direction difficult. Because some people are able to experience wide fluctuations in weight, however, the validity of this model is questioned. An alternative model, the _____ _____ model, assumes that positive reinforcement plays an important role in weight maintenance. Thus, people may overeat for a variety of reasons, including food preferences, cultural influences on eating and body composition, and availability of _____.

C. Is Obesity Unhealthy?

The question of obesity's effect on health depends on the method of measuring obesity, degree of obesity, _____ of weight, and history of weight cycling. The increased risks of obesity are largest for _____ disease and diabetes. Fat around the _____ is more of a risk than fat on the _____. Some research evidence indicates that gaining or losing weight is more _____ than maintaining a stable weight.

IV. Dieting

Dieting is not equally distributed among either overweight or normal weight people. By gender, the people most likely to diet are _____; by age, it is _____ people; and by socioeconomic status, it is people from the _____ and _____ - _____ classes.

A. Approaches to Losing Weight

Low-carbohydrate and high-fat diets tend to be popular because they do not restrict the amount of _____ and fat. Single-food diets, including liquid diets lead to weight loss due to greatly reduced _____ as people become progressively bored with the single food.   Behavior modification programs for weight control attempt to _____ healthy eating patterns and often included diet diaries, self-rewards, and penalties for cheating. One component of many diet programs is _____ because it speeds body metabolism, builds muscle, and improves the ratio of muscle to fat. Diet pills, fasting, and diets that allow fewer than 1,000 calories a day should be used only under _____ supervision.   As in treatment for smoking, problem drinking, and drug use, a major problem for weight loss programs is _____, because a majority of people who lose weight on any type of diet program will regain the lost weight.

B. Is Dieting Work a Good Choice?

Some experts recommend against dieting and counsel overweight people to concentrate on eating sensibly, _____ regularly, and maintaining their health. Periodic dieting may be a poor choice for older people, normal-weight people, and people who cannot attain their weight goals or whose weight

_____.

V. Eating Disorders

Besides overeating and cyclic dieting, two other eating disorders have been studied by health psychologists. Both anorexia nervosa and

_____ begin as attempts to control weight, and both may eventually produce dangerous physical effects.

A. Anorexia Nervosa

The eating disorder characterized by intentional self-starvation or semistarvation, sometimes to the point of death is called _____

_____. More than 90% of anorexics are _____;

most are young, European American, outwardly compliant, ambitious, and

_____ achievers. As weight loss continues, anorexics typically lose interest in sex, become hostile and irritable, constantly feel cold, grow a soft covering of body hair, lose scalp hair, and often develop a preoccupation with

_____. Even among high risk groups, such as adolescent girls in private schools, the prevalence of anorexia is less than _____ percent.

Motivation of anorexics to change eating habits and to gain weight is very

_____. Forced feeding usually restores _____, but it is not a cure.

B. Bulimia

Bulimia is the eating disorder in which people eat huge quantities of food in an uncontrolled manner (binge) and then get rid of the food by

_____ or using laxatives (purge). Compared with anorexics,

bulimics are likely to be older, less achievement oriented, abusers of alcohol,

aware that their eating habits are _____, filled with guilt, and

depressed. Like anorexics, most bulimics are _____. Bulimia

is almost never fatal, but eating large quantities of sweets can result in a

deficiency of sugar in the blood called _____ . Other

health consequences of frequent purging include: anemia, or inadequate

_____ _____ cells; electrolyte imbalance, and

alkalosis, an abnormally high level of alkaline in the body tissues. Unlike

anorexics, bulimics usually have _____ motivation to get better.

Answers

I.   mouth; peristalsis; small intestine; liver; large intestine; decreases; hunger
II.   physical activity (exercise)
II.A. metabolism; losing; obsessed
II.B. unpleasant; difficult
III.   calories; obesity
III.A. body fat; body mass; obesity
III.B. setpoint; positive incentive; food
III.C. distribution; heart (cardiovascular); middle (stomach); hips (thighs); dangerous (unhealthy)
IV.   women; young; middle; upper-middle
IV.A. protein; calories; reinforce (reward); exercise; medical; relapse
IV.B. exercising; fluctuates
V.   bulimia
V.A.. anorexia nervosa; female (women); high; food; 1; low; weight
V.B.   vomiting; abnormal (harmful); women; hypoglycemia; red blood; high (strong)

Multiple Choice Questions

_____ 1. Which of these statements is typical of most anorexics?
a. They have been thin throughout their lives.
b. They experience large cycles of weight gain and loss.
c. They exercise vigorously for long periods of time.
d. They frequently steal food and other items.

_____ 2. Which of these statements is typical of most bulimics?
a. They are usually younger than anorexics.
b. They exercise vigorously for long periods of time.
c. They are usually thinner than anorexics.
d. They use laxatives and vomiting as a means of weight control.

_____ 3. Peristalsis is
a. the first step in the digestive process.
b. the rhythmic contraction and relaxation of muscles that propel food through the digestive system.
c. the exchange of gases across the alveoli.
d. both a and b

_____ 4. During World War II, a team of researchers found that normal young men changed their behavior, began to exhibit irritability and aggression, lost interest in sex and other activities, and became preoccupied with food. These young men were showing the effects of
a. amphetamine use.
b. living in a prison camp.
c. experimental overfeeding.
d. semistarvation.

_____ 5. Campbell's weight is 20 pounds below normal as a result of 2 months of a 600-calorie-a-day diet. You would expect that Campbell will
a. feel more energetic than usual.
b. become disinterested in food.
c. be constantly hungry.
d. not be able to regain is normal weight even after he increases his food intake to 3200 calories a day.

_____ 6. Being overweight
a. has a survival advantage during times of food shortages.
b. greatly decreases one's energy level.
c. is solely a matter of heredity.
d. all of the above

_____ 7. Unlike weight charts, the waist-to-hip ratio measures
   a. the distribution of body fat.
   b. level of obesity.
   c. total weight.
   d. inheritability of obesity.

_____ 8. The definition of body mass index includes
   a. body build.
   b. age.
   c. gender.
   d. height and weight.
   e. all of the above

_____ 9. The notion that people have a type of internal thermostat that regulates how much they weigh is called
   a. the glucostatic mechanism.
   b. the setpoint concept.
   c. adipose range.
   d. the lipostatic mechanism.

_____ 10. Which of these statements is most consistent with the positive incentive model?
   a. People eat primarily to store calories for times when food is not plentiful.
   b. People have a biologically determined weight and will have difficulty deviating from that weight.
   c. A person who doesn't like hotdogs may eat them at a ball game when others are eating them.
   d. A person will eat huge quantities of food in an effort to resolve inner conflict.

_____ 11. Which of these people has the HIGHEST risk of a weight-related health problem?
   a. a 19-year-old woman whose weight is 15% above that suggested by the weight chart.
   b. a middle-aged man who is 22 pounds overweight and whose weight is quite stable.
   c. a middle-aged man who is 22 pounds overweight, with most of the extra pounds distributed around his middle.
   d. a middle-age women who is 20 pounds overweight, with most of the extra pounds distributed around her hips and thighs.

_____ 12. Which of these groups of people is MOST likely to diet to lose weight?
   a. adolescent boys
   b. adolescent girls
   c. African American women
   d. European American men

_____ 13. People wanting to lose weight should
   a. avoid physical activity because it increases appetite.
   b. avoid exercise because it raises the setpoint.
   c. incorporate exercise into their daily routine.
   d. exercise regularly and eat a high calorie diet.

_____ 14. Very low calorie diets
   a. do not produce weight loss.
   b. can be nutritionally sound.
   c. have a serious problem with relapse.
   d. should not include exercise as part of one's routine.

_____ 15. Which group of people is MOST likely to decrease their level of obesity 10 years after dieting?
   a. middle-aged men
   b. middle-aged women
   c. young women
   d. children

_____ 16. Which of these weight-related factors is LEAST related to all-cause mortality for middle-aged European American women?
   a. a history of cycling weight gain and loss
   b. a waist-to-hip ratio of 0.75
   c. a body mass index of 40.0
   d. a history of being 10 to 12 pounds over ideal weight

_____ 17. When Marshall was a 21-year-old college junior, he was five feet-nine inches tall and weighed 155 pounds. Now at age 60, Marshall weighs 170 pounds. Thus, Marshall
   a. is at an elevated risk for mortality due to gaining 15 pounds.
   b. should diet until he weighs about 155 to 160 pounds.
   c. should diet until he weighs less than 150 pounds.
   d. he should not worry about the additional 15 pounds.
   e. both a and b

_____ 18. During the past 2 decades, the average U.S. adult has decreased dietary fat from 40% of energy intake to about 33%. During this time, the average U.S. adult has
   a. become fatter.
   b. become thinner due to increased exercise.
   c. become thinner due to this reduction in dietary fat.
   d. decreased sugar intake.

_____ 19. Some people who smoke say that they would like to quit, but they are afraid that they will gain weight. Which of these courses of action probably would have the MOST damaging health consequences?
   a. continue to smoke and maintain present weight
   b. quit smoking and gain 10 to 15 pounds
   c. quit smoking and gain 20 to 25 pounds
   d. quit smoking and maintain present weight

_____ 20. People with anorexia nervosa are most often
   a. middle-age women.
   b. European American male adolescents.
   c. European American female adolescents.
   d. African American female adolescents.

_____ 21. Anorexics are LEAST likely to
   a. see themselves as too thin.
   b. be preoccupied with food.
   c. be ambitious and perfectionistic.
   d. have hostile feelings toward their mother.

_____ 22. Which of these conditions is MOST characteristics of a person with bulimia?
   a. severely overweight
   b. severely underweight
   c. use of laxatives to purge
   d. amenorrhea

Multiple Choice Answers

1.	c	8.	d	15	d
2.	d	9.	b	16.	b
3.	b	10.	c	17.	d
4.	d	11.	c	18.	a
5.	c	12.	b	19.	a
6.	a	13.	c	20.	c
7.	a	14.	c	21.	a
				22.	c

Essay Questions

1. Loraine is 15 pounds overweight and is concerned about her health because of the 15 pounds. Loraine believes that she needs to go on a diet to lose the weight as quickly as possible. Is she correct about the health implications of her extra pounds, and what type of diet should she avoid?

2. You receive a case report of a young woman with an eating disorder, but the report does not say whether she is anorexic or bulimic. What symptoms would you look for to determine which disorder she has?

Good points to include in your essay answers:

1. A. Loraine is probably incorrect in her belief that she needs to lose weight because of health concerns.
    1. There is a connection between obesity and several disorders.
    2. Loraine is not sufficiently overweight to put her at such risk.
    B. Loraine should avoid diets that:
    1. Will lead to rapid weight loss.
    2. Are very low in carbohydrates and high in fat because these diets are not effective and can endanger health.
    3. Consist of a single food because these diets are boring, difficult to continue, and nutritional disasters.
    4. Consist of less than 1,000 calories per day because these diets are nutritionally risky.
    5. Rely on drugs to suppress her appetite.

2. A. Some symptoms would not allow you to determine the difference.
    1. She would probably exhibit a great concern with weight if she had anorexia or bulimia.
    2. She would probably be secretive about her eating habits with either disorder.
    B. To determine if the young woman was anorexic or bulimic, you might look for:
    1. A difference in eating; anorexics refrain from eating whereas bulimics binge eat.
    2. Her to be very thin if she were anorexic and of normal weight if she were bulimic.
    3. Self-restraint if she were anorexic and impulsiveness if she were bulimic.
    4. Feelings of self-satisfaction and euphoric if she were anorexic and feelings of depression and guilt if she were bulimic.
    5. Dental problems that would signal bulimia.
    6. A lack of willingness to be in treatment if she were anorexic and a willingness to be in treatment if she were bulimic.

Let's Get Personal—
Analyzing Your Eating

To better understand your eating patterns, keep a food diary for at least a week. Record when you eat, the types of food and beverages, and estimated portion sizes. Choose a typical week to keep your record, and try not to change your eating. Don't cheat—you won't be able to understand your eating if you make changes or fail to report honestly. The goal of keeping the food diary is to get information so that you can analyze how healthy your diet and eating patterns are.

Day 1		Day 2	
Breakfast	Time:	Breakfast	Time:
Snack	Time:	Snack	Time:
Lunch	Time:	Lunch	Time:
Snack	Time:	Snack	Time:
Dinner	Time:	Dinner	Time:
Snack	Time:	Snack	Time:

Day 3

Breakfast   Time:

_____

_____

_____

Snack   Time:

_____

Lunch   Time:

_____

_____

_____

Snack   Time:

_____

Dinner   Time:

_____

_____

_____

Snack   Time:

_____

Day 4

Breakfast   Time:

_____

_____

_____

Snack   Time:

_____

Lunch   Time:

_____

_____

_____

Snack   Time:

_____

Dinner   Time:

_____

_____

_____

Snack   Time:

_____

Day 5

Breakfast   Time:

_____

_____

_____

Snack   Time:

_____

Lunch   Time:

_____

_____

_____

Snack   Time:

_____

Dinner   Time:

_____

_____

_____

Snack   Time:

_____

Day 6

Breakfast   Time:

_____

_____

_____

Snack   Time:

_____

Lunch   Time:

_____

_____

_____

Snack   Time:

_____

Dinner   Time:

_____

_____

_____

Snack   Time:

_____

Day 7

Breakfast Time:	Dinner Time:
_____	_____
_____	_____
_____	_____

Snack Time:	Snack Time:
_____	_____

Lunch   Time:

_____

_____

_____

Snack   Time:

_____

Did anything surprise you about your eating?

Do you eat more than you had imagined?

Do you eat more "junk foods" than you thought?

Do you skip meals, either in an attempt to diet or because you have little time?

Did skipping meals result in snacking or unwise choices after a skipped meal?

CHAPTER 16
Exercising

Fill in the Rest of the Story

I. Types of Exercise

Nearly all types of exercise can be grouped under one of five basic kinds of physical activity, each of which may contribute to strength, flexibility, speed, or physical fitness. The type of exercise that involves contracting muscles against an immovable object is called _____ exercise. Weight lifting and some forms of calisthenics that require muscle contraction and joint movement qualify as isotonic exercise, which can build _____ strength and endurance and improve body appearance. The type of exercise that requires specialized equipment that adjusts the amount of resistance according to the amount of force applied is called _____ exercise. Fast, short-distance running, such as sprinting in track or running the bases in baseball, would be considered as _____ exercise. Aerobic exercise requires greatly increased _____ consumption over an extended time and can be achieved through walking, jogging, swimming, dancing, bicycling, and several other activities. Aerobic exercise benefits both the respiratory system and the _____ system.

II. Reasons for Exercising

People who exercise list a number of reasons for their activity, including physical fitness, _____ control, and cardiorespiratory fitness.

A. Physical Fitness

Fitness can be considered as either *organic* or *dynamic*. The type of fitness that refers to inherited characteristics is called _____, whereas _____ fitness is determined by the amount and kinds of exercise a person performs. The five basic types of exercise can contribute to muscle strength, muscle _____ , flexibility, and cardiorespiratory fitness. Cardiorespiratory fitness can only be accomplished through _____ exercise.

B. Weight Control

Exercise combined with _____ is an excellent way to lose weight, but exercise alone is sufficient to lower the ratio of _____ tissue to muscle tissue and thus improve body composition. Exercise alone does not burn many _____, but exercise performed at least four times a week does seem to elevate _____ rate, which in turn helps control weight.

III. Cardiovascular Effects of Exercise

More important than physical fitness or weight control is the issue of exercise and _____ health.

A. Early Studies

During the early 1950s, studies found that sedentary workers were more prone to _____ disease than were active workers. Ralph

Paffenbarger and his colleagues investigated physical activity and health in a group of San Francisco longshoremen and found that CHD death rates were more than 80% higher for _____ - _____ workers than for the high-activity ones. Paffenbarger also studied Harvard alumni and found that the least active men had a much increased of heart attack compared with the most active ones. In general, the Harvard alumni study found that men who expended 2,000 kcal or more per week can expect an average increase in longevity of about _____ years. Exercise in excess of that level does not seem to add any more protection against heart attack. The main limitation of Paffenbarger's studies was their exclusive use of _____ participants.

B. Later Studies

Studies over the past 20 years have tended to measure all physical activity, both on and off the _____ and to include _____ as participants. The Framingham Heart Study followed a large number of women and men over a long period but failed to find evidence that exercise protected against heart disease for _____ largely because most of these participants were quite similar in level of physical activity. At the extremes of activity, however, very inactive women were more than twice as likely to develop heart disease than the most active women, suggesting that a _____ lifestyle can be dangerous for women as well as for men. The Alameda County Study found that both women and men can _____ life span through leisure-time physical activity.

Results from these and other more recent studies suggest that people can reduce

their _____ _____ index, improve waist-to-hip ratio, and

increase longevity.

C. Exercise and Stroke

Physical activity seems to offer _____ protection against

stroke than it does against heart disease, especially for _____

American men. In general, however, the effects of exercise are not as dramatic

for stroke as they are for _____ disease.

D. Exercise and Cholesterol Levels

One possibility for the protective effect of exercise is through increases in

_____ - _____ lipoprotein. Research indicates that

aerobic exercise can raise HDL levels without affecting _____ -

_____ lipoprotein levels, resulting in a more favorable ratio of

_____ _____ to HDL.

IV. Other Health Benefits of Physical Activity

Some evidence suggests that physical activity offers some protection

against some types of cancer and loss of _____ density. In addition,

exercise may be able to control of diabetes and confer _____

benefits, such as decreased depression, reduced anxiety, and increased self-

esteem.

A. Physiological Benefits

More specifically, research indicates that regular physical activity may

reduce colon cancer and _____ cancer in men, and may offer

women some protection against _____ cancer. Exercise also

protects women and men against _____, a disease caused by

loss of calcium. Both pre- and postmenopausal women can gain protection

against loss of _____ _____ by regular physical

activity. Physical activity may be a useful weapon in the control of adult-onset

_____, and research also shows that exercise is an important

component in managing _____ - _____ diabetes.

Findings from one study suggested that when older men and women with sleep

difficulties began a program of brisk walking, they significantly

_____ their sleep problems.

B. Psychological Benefits of Exercise

Research indicates that people who participate in an aerobic exercise

program receive such psychological benefits as decreased depression, reduced

anxiety, less stress, and increased _____- _____. In

general, both aerobic and _____ exercise can reduce depression in

both normal and _____ populations. Also, regular physical activity

is probably at least as effective as _____ in treating depression.

In addition, physical activity is especially effective in reducing

_____ anxiety, that is, a temporary experience of anxiety due to a specific situation. Moreover, exercise seems to buffer the negative effects of _____, but evidence is lacking that aerobic exercise can prevent stress-related illness. People who exercise regularly often have positive feelings about their body shape and physical health, which may contribute to their feelings of high _____ - _____.

V. Hazards of Physical Activity

Although its benefits are numerous, a regular physical activity program is also associated with some potential dangers.

A. Exercise Addiction

Some people become so dependent on exercise that it interferes with other parts of their lives. Nevertheless, research does not support the idea that exercise causes the release of _____, a necessary condition for addiction. The Commitment to Exercise Scale measures the two factors of Obligatory and _____ exercisers who continue to exercise in the face of adverse circumstances, such as injuries, or who permit their activity to take precedence over other aspects of their lives.

B. Injuries from Physical Activity

Regular exercisers are also at risk for a variety of injuries, but _____ injury is the most common. Injuries are most frequent among _____ exercisers, such as "weekend athletes."

C. Death during Exercise

Death during exercise is _____ likely than during other

times, so a medical checkup is a wise precaution for older, unfit, sedentary

people who want to begin an exercise program.

VI. How Much Is Enough but not Too Much?

In recent years, many experts have come to view exercise as a subset of

_____ _____ and have emphasized the benefit of

_____ rather than prolonged or strenuous activity. Experts

now recommend that every adult should accumulate _____ minutes of

moderate physical activity a day, or at least on most days. More exercise may

improve endurance or body composition, but it may also increase the risk of

injuries without adding to _____ fitness.

VII. Maintaining a Physical Activity Program

Of all the people who begin a prescribed exercise program, about

_____ percent drop out within 6 months.

A. Predicting Dropouts

A number of factors are related to exercise dropouts, including low

motivation, depression, low self-efficacy, obesity, being a smoker, having a

_____-collar job, and having an inactive lifestyle. Conversely, the

people most likely to continue in a physical activity program are men, people

with a past history of physical activity, those with _____ levels

of education and income, and younger people.

B. Increasing Maintenance

Psychological programs increase exercise maintenance have included reinforcement for healthy behaviors, contracting, self-monitoring, instruction, modeling, goal setting, increased self-efficacy, and _____ prevention, These interventions increase maintenance rates by about 15% to 20%. Compliance to prescribed exercise programs can also be increased by building the patient's _____ support system.

Answers

I.   isometric; muscle; isokinetic; anaerobic; oxygen; circulatory (cardiovascular)
II.   weight
II.A.   organic; dynamic; endurance; aerobic
II.B.   diet; fat; calories; metabolic
III.   cardiovascular
III.A. heart (cardiovascular); low-activity; 2; male
III.B. job; women; sedentary (inactive); increase; body mass
III.C. less; African; heart
III.D. high-density; low-density; total cholesterol
IV.   bone; psychological
IV.A.   prostate; breast; osteoporosis; bone density; diabetes; juvenile-onset; decreased
IV.B.   self-esteem; nonaerobic; clinical, psychotherapy; trait; stress;self-esteem
V.A   endorphins; Pathological
V.B.   musculoskeletal; infrequent
V.C.   more
VI.   physical activity; moderate; 30; cardiovascular
VII.   50
VII.A. blue; higher
VII.B. relapse; social

Multiple Choice Questions

_____ 1. An example of isotonic exercise would be
   a. pushing hard against a solid wall.
   b. lifting weights.
   c. running 100 yards very quickly.
   d. jogging five miles.

_____ 2. The goal of isometric exercise is to
   a. increase cardiovascular fitness.
   b. increase muscle strength.
   c. reduce state anxiety.
   d. to increase oxygen intake.

_____ 3. An example of anaerobic exercise would be
   a. pushing hard against a solid wall.
   b. lifting weights.
   c. running 100 meters quickly.
   d. jogging five miles.

_____ 4. This type of exercise uses specialized equipment that adjusts the
   amount of resistance according to the amount of force applied, thus
   requiring exertion for lifting and additional effort for returning to the
   starting position.
   a. isokinetic
   b. isotonic
   c. isometric
   d. anaerobic
   e. aerobic

_____ 5. An example of aerobic exercise would be
   a. pushing hard against a sold wall.
   b. lifting weights.
   c. running 100 yards quickly.
   d. jogging five miles.

_____ 6. Randall has always wanted to be an outstanding athlete, but he has
   little natural ability. Nevertheless, Randall has worked hard and is
   currently a distance runner at his university. Randall now has
   a. organic fitness.
   b. dynamic fitness.
   c. both of the above.
   d. neither a nor b

_____ 7. Aerobic fitness is negatively related to
    a. cardiorespiratory fitness.
    b. risk of heart disease.
    c. organic fitness.
    d. muscle flexibility.

_____ 8. People who lose weight through exercise do so mostly because
    a. exercise burns calories at a fast rate.
    b. exercise diminishes appetite and thus decreases food consumption.
    c. exercise elevates metabolism.
    d. people who wish to exercise tend to diet in order to improve their appearance in exercise clothes.

_____ 9 Your friend Clayton is a sedentary, slightly overweight smoker who asks you for advice on quitting smoking. He is worried that he may gain too much weight if he quits. What advice should you give him?
    a. Quit smoking, go on a very low calorie diet, and then begin a regular physical activity program.
    b. Quit smoking, eat regularly, and begin a program of physical activity that gradually builds up to about 3 hours a week.
    c. Quit smoking, begin a 1,000 calorie a day diet, and engage in isometric exercise 2 to 3 hours a week.
    d. Continue to smoke because some people who quit gain 40 to 50 pounds.

_____ 10. The Harvard alumni study found that
    a. physical activity reduced one's risk of heart attack but did not increase length of life.
    b. exercise equivalent to jogging 20 miles per week decreased the risk of heart attack.
    c. exercise equivalent to jogging 40 miles per week decreased the risk of heart attack significantly more than 20 miles per week.
    d. exercise increased length of life but did not reduce risk of heart attack.

_____ 11 Researchers have found that physical activity is most likely to protect against stroke in
    a. middle-age and elderly men.
    b. elderly women.
    c. African American women of all ages.
    d. middle-age women.
    e. smokers of all ages.

_____ 12. Research evidence is strongest in support of the hypothesis that exercise protects against heart disease by
   a. increasing HDL.
   b. decreasing HDL.
   c. increasing LDL.
   d. decreasing LDL.

_____ 13. For people interested in lowering their risk of heart disease,
   a. exercise is a valuable component in a program designed to lower risk factors.
   b. exercise alone is protective and allows less attention to diet and other risk factors.
   c. exercise will confer immunity against heart disease.
   d. exercise is more of a risk than a benefit.

_____ 14. Evidence is strong that physical activity protects against cardiovascular disease. Additional evidence indicates that exercise protects against
   a. lung cancer.
   b. skin cancer.
   c. colon cancer.
   d. unintentional injuries.

_____ 15. Women ages 50 to 70 who begin an exercise program are likely to
   a. gain bone mineral density.
   b. lose bone mineral density.
   c. develop osteoporosis.
   d. retain bone mineral density.

_____ 16 In general, a physical activity program is likely to
   a. increase depression in clinically depressed people.
   b. decrease depression clinically depressed people.
   c. increase depression in nonclinically depressed people.
   d. decrease depression in nonclinically depressed people.
   e. both b and d

_____ 17. Research suggest that anxiety can be lowered by
   a. aerobic exercise.
   b. isotonic exercise (weight lifting).
   c. both a and b
   d. neither a nor b

_____ 18. Camey wishes to lower her high level of state anxiety. Which activity would you recommend?
   a. jogging
   b. relaxation training
   c. transcendental meditation
   d. any activity that provides a change of pace

_____ 19. Lee is quite dependent on exercise, running 10 to 15 miles every day and allowing running to interfere with his job and family life. You would guess that Lee
   a. has a physiological addiction to running.
   b. is an ex-college athlete who is trying to relive past achievements.
   c. has low expectations of himself.
   d. is overly concerned about his weight and physical appearance.

_____ 20. Research indicates that death during exercise
   a. is more likely for people who are usually sedentary but who engage in occasional vigorous exercise.
   b. is not possible for physically fit individuals.
   c. occurs more for people who have a regular aerobic program than for people who exercise anaerobically once a week.
   d. is less likely than death while watching television.

_____ 21. Fernando is a 24-year-old banker who is 25 pounds overweight and who wants to begin an exercise program to lose weight. You would advise him to
   a. begin by jogging four or five miles a day, six days a week.
   b. keep repeating to himself, "No pain, no gain."
   c. weigh himself every day to document the effectiveness of his exercise program.
   d. begin slowly and gradually work up to 3 or 4 hours of moderate physical activity six or seven days a week.

_____ 22. Experts currently recommend that
   a. people with a history of heart problems avoid hard physical activity.
   b. adults accumulate 30 minutes of moderate physical activity a day or at least on most days.
   c. children benefit from moderate exercise but adults do not.
   d. adults benefit from moderate exercise but children do not.

Multiple Choice Answers

1.	b	12.	a
2.	b	13.	a
3.	c	14.	c
4.	a	15.	d
5.	d	16.	e
6 .	b	17.	c
7	b	18.	d
8 .	c	19.	d
9 .	b	20.	a
10.	b	21.	d
11.	a	22.	b

Essay Questions

1. Evaluate the statement, "It takes too much exercise to burn off the calories in this ice cream bar. I'd be better off just skipping the ice cream and not having to do the exercise."

2. Graham is a 35-year-old accountant who started running as a way to control his weight and improve his cardiovascular health. He now runs over 80 miles a week. Is his program helping or harming his health?

Good points to include in your essay answers:

1. A. Exercise alone does not expend many calories but
        1. Exercise alone can produce weight loss.
        2. Exercise may raise the metabolic level and may possibly adjust the body's setpoint, allowing permanent weight loss.
    B. Exercise is a beneficial component in an weight loss or weight maintenance program.
        1. Physical activity is a factor in the weight-maintenance equation, increasing the number of calories expended and building muscle tissue.
        2. Exercise can help maintain lean body mass in moderate-weight exercisers.

2. A. Graham's exercise habits are probably both helping and harming his health.
    B. His cardiovascular health will probably benefit.
        1. Research shows that aerobic exercise has cardiovascular benefits, lowers the risk of several types of cancer, improves bone mineral density, decreases depression and anxiety, and is related to improved self-esteem.
        2. His exercise is far more strenuous than what is necessary for health benefits.
    C. His exercise habits pose risks.
        1. Graham may be addicted to exercise.
            a. He may neglect work, family, and other activities in order to run .
            b. He may ignore injury to continue running.
        2. The more miles run per week, the higher the chances of injury, putting Graham at risk.

Let's Get Personal—
Work Out

Do you get enough exercise but not too much? Exercise too little, and you fail to gain health benefits. Exercise too much, and you risk injury. Should you play a sport, lift weights, run, do aerobics, or some combination? Determining what is the right amount and right type of exercise is not easy.

Examine your exercise habits by answering the following questions:

Do you have an exercise program?

Does your exercising best fit the pattern of

    Activity at least 4 days a week

    Sedentary weekdays and active weekends

Circle the type or types of exercise you perform.

Isometric   Isotonic   Isokinetic   Anaerobic   Aerobic

How long are each of your exercise sessions?

Do you exercise enough to get optimal health benefits—that is, do you expend 2,000 kcal per week in cumulative energy expenditure?

What injuries have you sustained during the past 6 months as a result of exercise?

What health benefits do you believe that you get from your exercising?

CHAPTER 17

Future Challenges

Fill in the Rest of the Story

I. Healthier People

Americans are becoming increasingly health conscious, and this concern has appeared in national policy as well as in individual behavior. The concern is reflected in declining mortality rates of _____ disease, stroke, unintentional injuries, and more recently, cancer. National policy is reflected in *Healthy People 2000,* a report that sets both broad and specific goals. The broad goals include increasing the span of _____ life, reducing health disparities among Americans, and achieving access to _____ services for all people in the United States.

A. Increasing the Span of Healthy Life

Increasing the span of healthy life is different from increasing life _____. A healthy life means being free from dysfunction, disease symptoms, and health-related problems. Each year of healthy life is called a _____ year.

B. Reducing Health Disparities

The United States does a _____ job of dispensing health care to its citizens than any other industrialized nation. African Americans,

Hispanic Americans, and _____ Americans have lower income and educational levels than European Americans and _____ Americans, and these disparities related to poorer access to health services, more risky behaviors, fewer health-protective behaviors, and shorter _____ _____.

C. Increasing Access to Preventive Services

Different types of prevention produce different levels of savings. Programs that keep people healthy by encouraging immunizations and lifestyle changes are considered as _____ prevention, and these programs tend to be good bargains. Secondary prevention programs include screening _____ - _____ people to discover disease in its early and more treatable stages, and these programs may not always be cost effective.

II. The Profession of Health Psychology

Health psychology can contribute to health by accumulating information on factors that relate to health and illness, promoting and maintaining health, preventing and treating illness, and formulating health policy and promoting the _____ _____ system.

A. Progress in Health Psychology

During the past 2 decades, the profession of health psychology has changed the field of psychology and has provided job opportunities for psychologists trained as health psychologists. These women and men work as clinicians, teachers, and _____ in settings that include universities,

_____ schools, and hospitals.

B. The Training of Health Psychologists

Health psychologists receive a solid core of training at the

_____ level before continuing an additional two or more years of

training in a variety of health-related subjects.

C. The Work of Health Psychologists

Health psychologists work in a variety of settings and perform many

different functions. Much of their work is _____ in nature; that

is, health psychologists frequently work with a team of health professionals,

including physicians, nurses, physical therapists, and counselors.

III. Outlook for Health Psychology

Despite its rapid growth, health psychology continues to face several

challenges. One challenge the field has faced and met is acceptance by the public

and by the _____ profession.

A. Future Challenges for Health Care

Two important challenges that health psychology must meet are the

changing profile of _____ and the escalation of _____

_____ costs. Cardiovascular disease and _____ are

the two leading causes of death in the United States, while _____

_____ are the leading cause of death for young people. Health

Psychology can play an important role in changing unhealthy and risky behaviors that contribute to these leading causes of death. An additional challenge for health psychology is the rising costs of health care, which have increased at a much higher rate than _____.

B. A Note of Cautious Optimism

Evan Pattishall has proposed two rules of caution that apply to health psychologists: First, "Don't propose more than you have _____ to support" and second, "Don't _____ more than you can deliver." Health psychology has followed this advice.

Answers

I.   heart (cardiovascular; healthy; preventive
I.A.   expectancy; well
I.B.   poorer; Native; Asian; life span
I.C.   primary; at-risk
II.   health care
II.A.   researchers; medical
II.B.   doctoral
II.C.   collaboraative
III.   medical
III.A.   illness; health care; cancer; unintentional injuries; inflation
III.B.   data; promise

Multiple Choice Questions

_____ 1. During the past 3 decades, the people of the United States have
   a. increased the amount of saturated fat in their diets.
   b. increased the rated of death from unintentional injuries.
   c. decreased their use of seatbelts and airbags.
   d. decreased their consumption of alcohol.

_____ 2. At age 65, women in the United States have another 19 years of life expectancy and about _____ years of health expectancy.
   a. 5
   b. 10
   c. 15
   d. 22

_____ 3. Compared with other industrialized countries, the United States ranks _____ in dispensing health care to its citizens.
   a. first
   b. third
   c. seventh
   d. last

_____ 4. Compared with African Americans, European Americans have
   a. a longer life expectancy.
   b. a higher infant mortality rate.
   c. an increased risk of death from cardiovascular disease.
   d. an increased risk of death from homicide.

_____ 5. Among Hispanic Americans, these people have the most education and the greatest likelihood of adequate health care and physician visits:
   a. Haitian Americans.
   b. Puerto Rican Americans.
   c. Mexican Americans.
   d. Cuban Americans.

_____ 6. Socioeconomic status has a strong influence on receiving health care in the United States. However, when socioeconomic factors are adjusted, this group has a high rate of risky behaviors and a low rate of receiving health services:
   a. Asian Americans.
   b. Native Americans.
   c. Cuban Americans.
   d. European Americans.

_____ 7. An example of secondary prevention would be
     a. early screening of people at risk for breast cancer.
     b. smoking prevention programs in elementary schools.
     c. improving the training of physicians, nurses, and other medical personnel.
     d. treating cancer patients with chemotherapy.

_____ 8. In the United States, the leading cause of death among people under 65 years of age is
     a. cancer.
     b. heart disease.
     c. stroke.
     d. AIDS.

_____ 9. In the United States, the leading cause of death for people between the ages of 15 and 24 is
     a. cancer.
     b. AIDS.
     c. unintentional injuries.
     d. homicide.
     e. suicide.

_____ 10. Health psychologists are most involved with
     a. treating illnesses.
     b. contributing to people's span of life.
     c. determining the causes of disease.
     d. decreasing the incidence of psychological disorders.
     e. adding healthy years to people's lives.

Answers

1.	d	6.	b
2.	b	7.	a
3.	d	8.	a
4.	a	9.	c
5.	d	10.	e

Essay Question

1. A friend of yours (who is a psychology major but who has not taken health psychology) tells you, "I don't want to be a health psychologist because I don't want to work with sick people in a hospital." Is her assessment correct in its description of the work done by health psychologists?